I0830419

So, we are born and are
given a life to make the
most of. But, in some cases,
and in one fell swoop, it can
all be taken away. In that
split second, for some it's
the end of the road. But
others get given a second
chance. Surgery. While
being given that second
chance, it is touch and go as
to that day is your last day,
or whether you appear back
in the room.

I was a ticking time bomb
and, in all fairness, was
given a few indicators along
the way until it was
confirmed I had a leaky
heart valve. It had worked
its hardest for many years
but suddenly was in need of
assistance.

This book is my story, and
the story of a few others
who have also experienced
heart surgery.

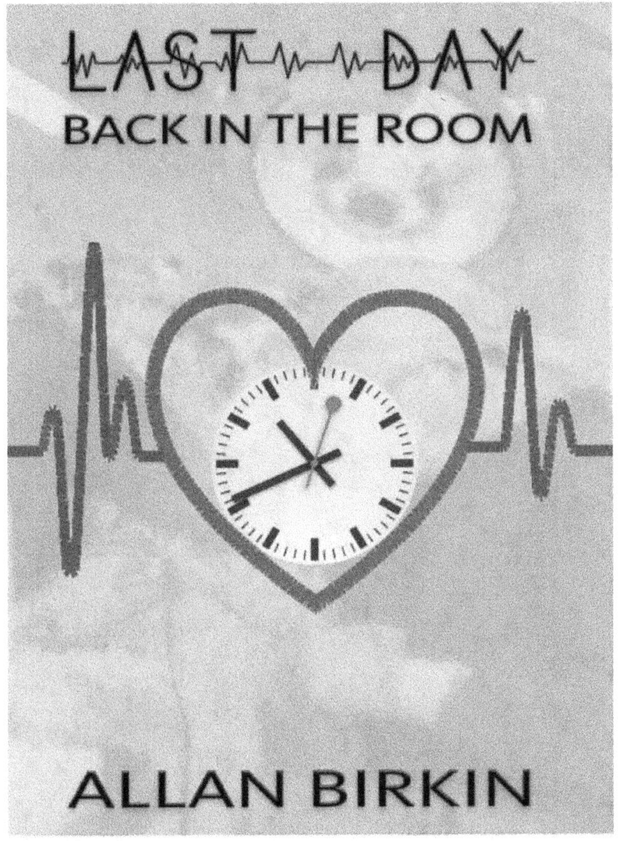

I've said before that two heads are better than one. This time, I got my dear friend, Tony Martin, to help design the front and back cover. I also insisted that he keep his feature of alternative front cover so in this book he gets a double whammy. All the best to you, my good friend,
Mr Anthony Martin.

TITLES TO DATE

Missed the Boat

Last Day Back in the Room

BY
ALLAN BIRKIN

ALLAN BIRKIN

LAST DAY
BACK IN THE
ROOM

www.wordsarelife.co.uk
A13 OMS PRESS

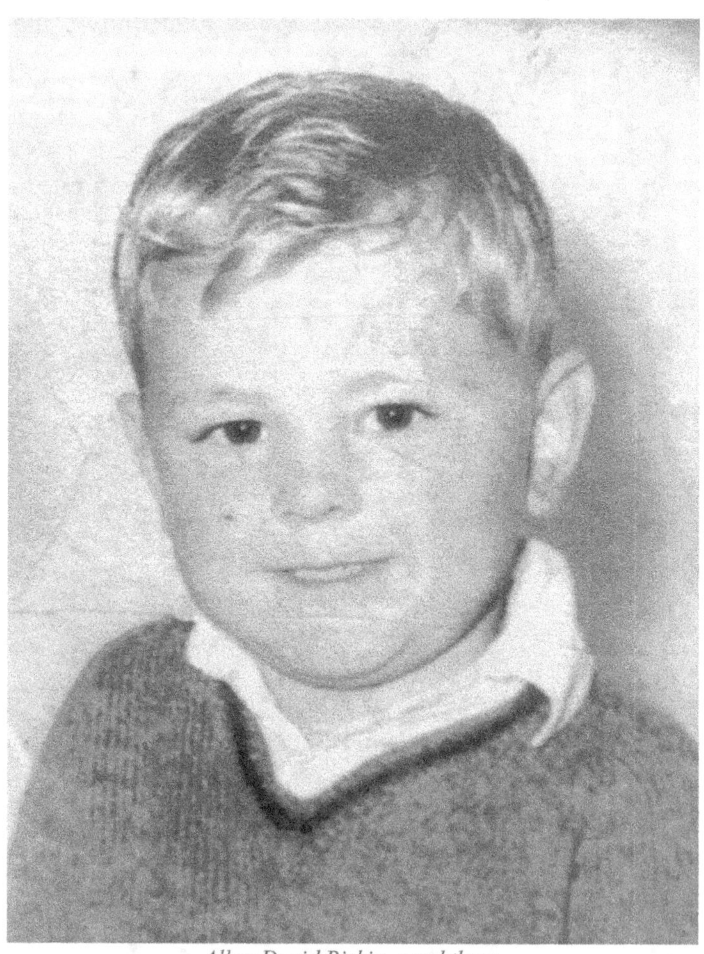

Allan David Birkin, aged three.

LAST DAY
BACK IN THE ROOM

ALLAN
BIRKIN

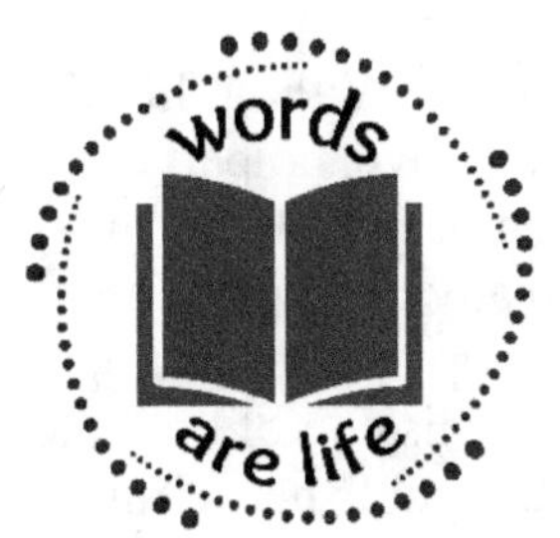

A 13 OMS PRESS

*** Salford *** Manchester *** United Kingdom***

FOR ALL WHO CARE TO READ

First published in Great Britain in 2023 by
Words Are Life
10 Chester Place,
Adlington, Chorley,
PR6 9RP

lesley@wordsarelife.co.uk

Available for purchase on Amazon.

Copyright (c) Allan Birkin and Words Are Life.

A13 OMS PRESS

Cover photograph: Shani Birkin Hodson
Back page cover: Allan, Shani, Ashley and Allan Jnr.
The Amateur Furrytographer since 1971.

LAST DAY BACK IN THE ROOM

So, no judgements please, just read it and enjoy! Rest assured. One thing is for sure. No monies will be returned to my coffers for this little read. All monies raised and donations received will go straight to the big tin that sits on the desk of the heart charity, the Ticker Club, based at Wythenshawe Hospital.

2
FOREWORD

ALLAN DAVID BIRKIN WAS born the 18th of September, 1960. The size and time will, unfortunately have to remain unknown, or just a little secret.

The son of Margaret Cooper, and (apparently) Allan Birkin – a man I met just the once in my life time and was destined never to meet again. This is because he's no longer roaming the planet, but also (and most important) because I have no desire to.

The man who is believed to be my biological father may just as well have been a stranger who walked by me in the street. He meant nothing to me, never would and never will.

At 19, I was a curious teenager who just had to get out of his system the curiosity of knowing who my biological dad was meant to be.

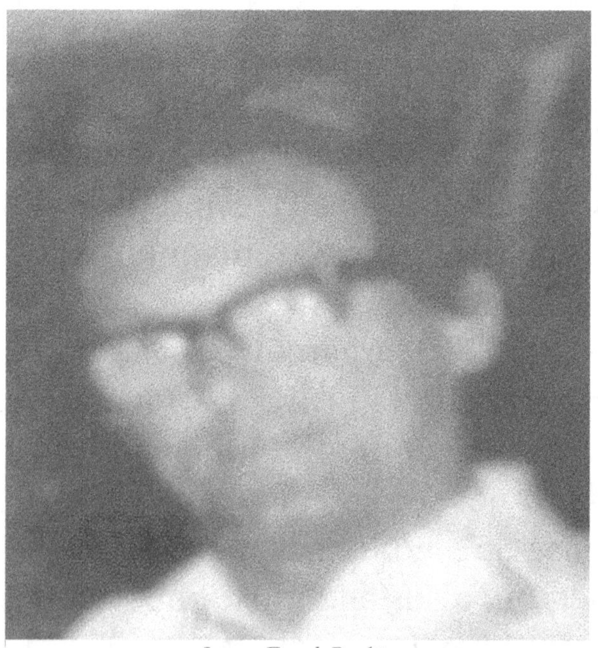

James Frank Parkin.

It was a decision I did live to regret. My father who brought me up for as long as I can remember was so upset, but it was something I just had to do.

James Frank Parkin was and always will be remembered as my father. He was a guy I have a lot of admiration for. He was a true gentleman and was taken from us all at far too young an age (49). Gone Friday May 24th 1984.

That man only ever raised his hand once to me. The one and only time he did was, believe you me, fully deserved. Not only that once, but probably a lot more. It is definitely true what they say. The good really do die young. Bless that man.

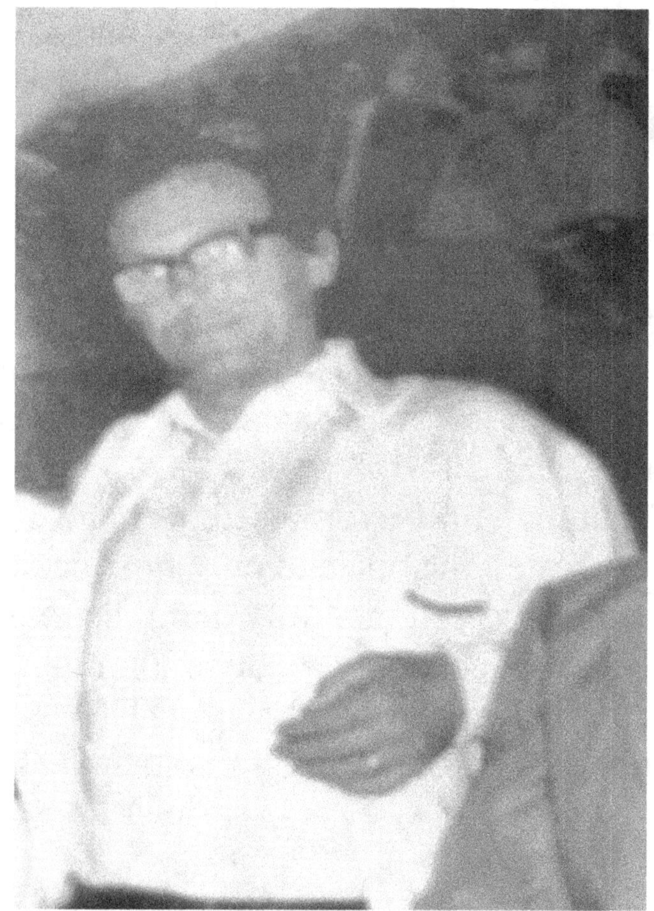

James Frank Parkin.

<u>3</u>
FALSE START

BINGO. AS THE RAIN begins to pour down outside, I finally put pen to paper and make a start. After all, I've been putting off till tomorrow what should have happened yesterday. Well, at least three months ago.

So today is here and off we go. Where do I start? Well, let me tell you this. Where I am going to start is not part of the original plan.

My opening line was meant to be "So, I heard it on the television" but instead I'm beginning with RIP Rick Grantham. I can't believe he's no longer with us.

As part of a bunch of mates who are all getting old, it we'd talk about (but not in a morbid way) which one of us would pop our clogs first. Never in a million years did any of us think it would be Rick. He was so laid back. In fact, if he was any slower, he would have stopped.

We all lost our bet, except Rex, of course. No way would he have bet on himself (haha) and we all bet on him! Little did Rick or any of us think it would be Rick who was our ticking time bomb!

I will never forget Tony Darcy ringing me up. He said, "I've got some bad news, mate". There was a pause, then out came the words that I can still hear today. "Rick's dead".

You often know when someone is ill, and they are dying. It becomes expected and allows you to get a little used to what's about to occur, but for it to happen out of the blue like that was like being hit in the face with a shovel. I couldn't believe it. In fact, I still can't. Rick, my friend of almost 30 years was gone in a split second. It's even harder for the other lads as they were even closer to Rick than I was. Apparently, he had completely blocked arteries and knew nothing of it apart from the fact he blamed everything on indigestion.

"What have you done to your ankle, Rick?" "Oh, it's indigestion," haha. And why would his first heart attack see him rushed to hospital in an ambulance for emergency stent surgery when a 2nd more powerful heart attack got him before the doctors had the chance to help. Our friend, Rick, was gone. He loved his overtime, the computer, his music and of course, not forgetting the wonderful ladies he left behind, his beautiful wife,

Susan, and their two much-loved daughters, Rachel and Kimberley who have been left to pick up the pieces and face a life without the man they all loved so much.

Testament to my fondness of the man, I still have umpteen CDs and MP3s he copied for me. it was for a small fee, of course, but I was ever so grateful and as long as I remain on this planet so will the metal silver box that contains those precious-to-me items. Nobody has copied me CDs ever since and nor will they either. We now live in era where CDs are becoming ever more extinct by the day. "Alexa, play me this" and "Play me that", but my CDs will stay as a reminder of a very, very nice man.

God bless you, buddy.

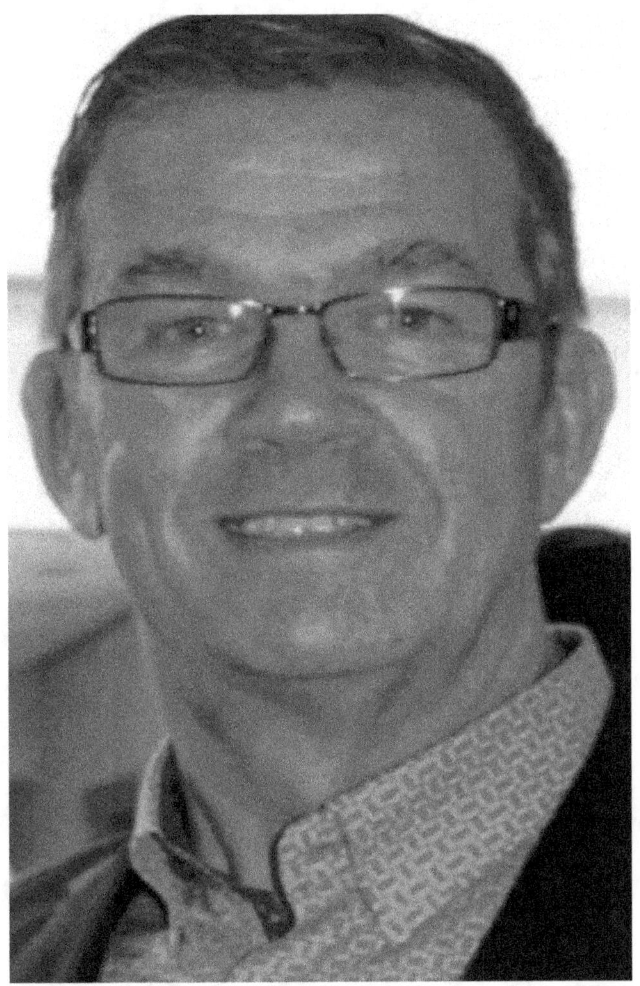

RIP Richard Grantham,
24 March 1960 - 15 July 2015.

I'm sad to say that, while writing this book, we have lost a few more of our friends:
David Regan (aka Rex),
David Harrison,
Steve Hindley,
Steve Corfield (aka Corky) and
Phil Lally.

Bless them all.

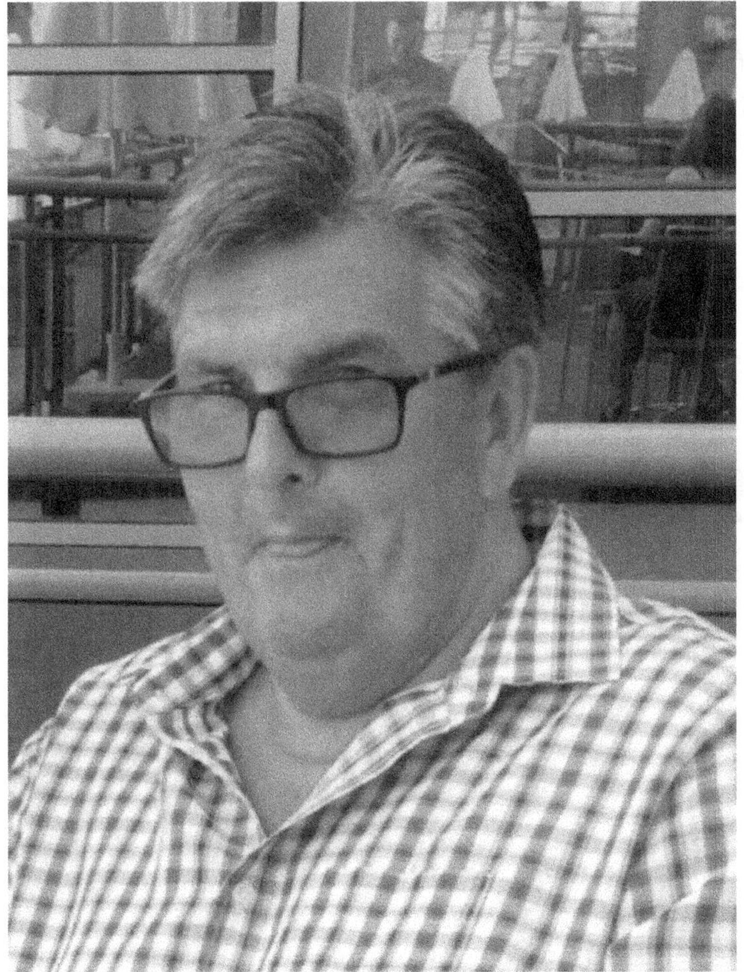

David Regan (aka Rex).

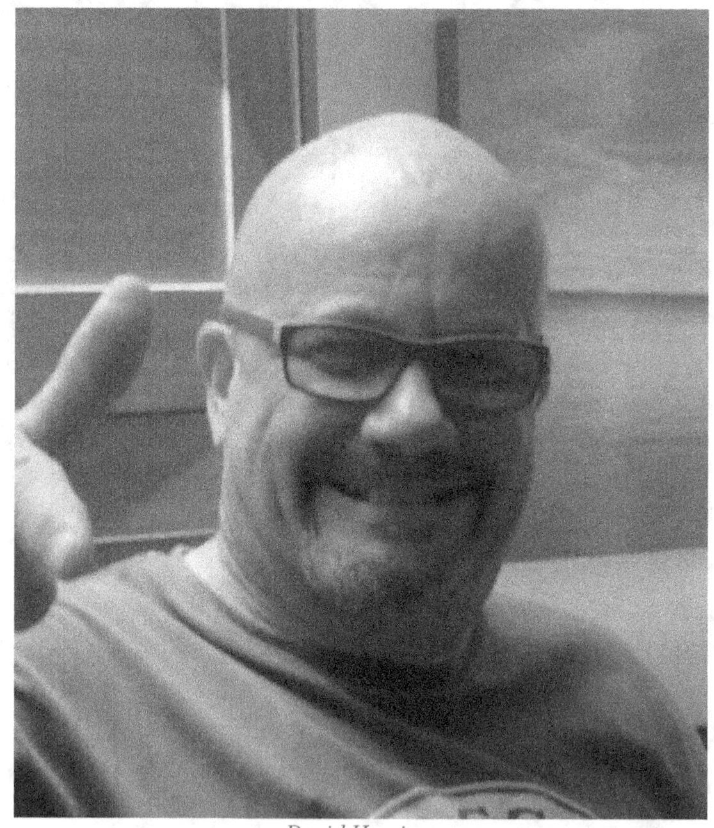

David Harrison

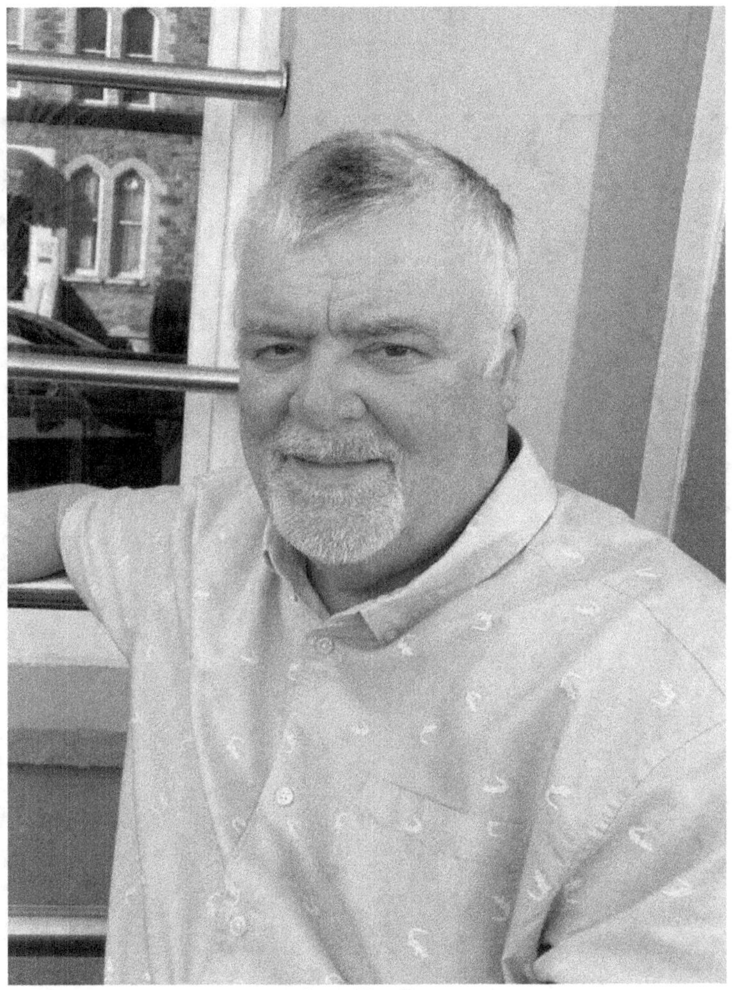

Steve Hindley.

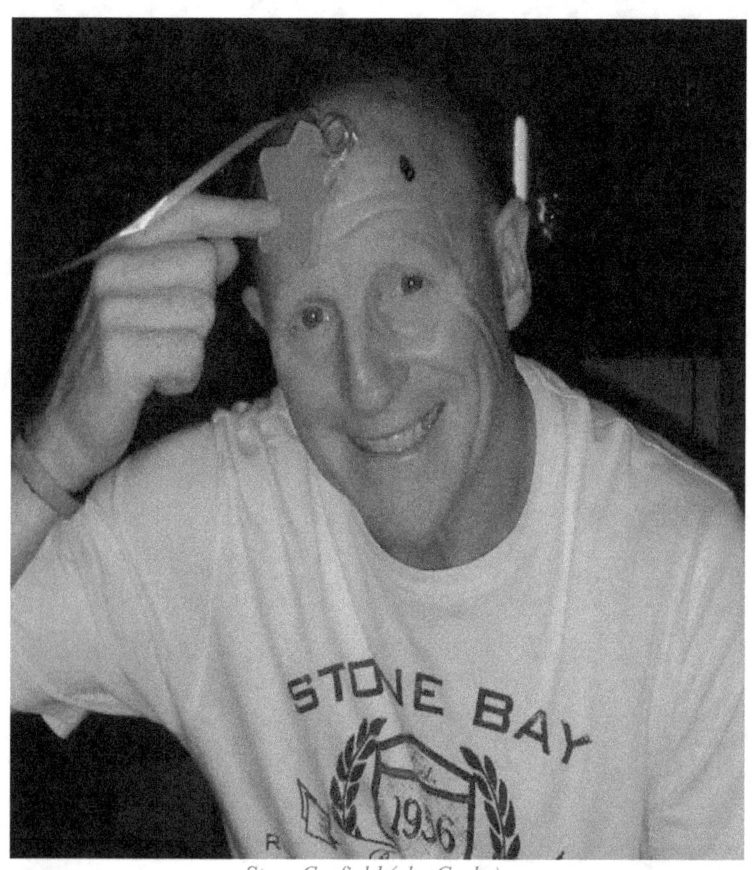

Steve Corfield (aka Corky)

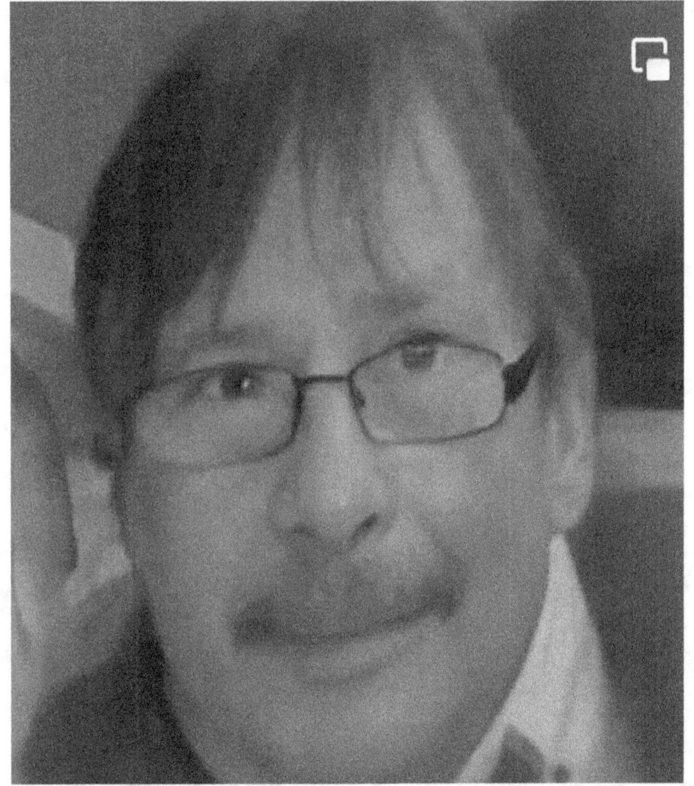

Phil Lally.

$\underline{4}$
THE START

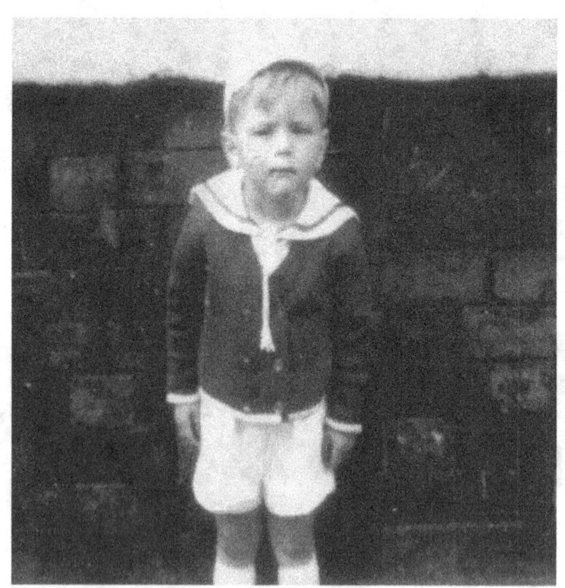

Allan in a sailor suit.

WELL, I'VE NEVER BEEN what you'd call an elite athlete, though I've competed in most sports. Whatever it is or was, you could be rest assured I'd give it my all.

Football, 5-a-side, 11-a-side, rugby, cricket, basketball, cross country... But I especially loved the 1500 metres, athletics, swimming, snooker, pool, darts, and even bastard dominoes, bowling, go-karting and cards, haha.

I'd have a go at any type of sport and give it my best shot. I always wanted to win. I played for the school football team in all three schools I attended.

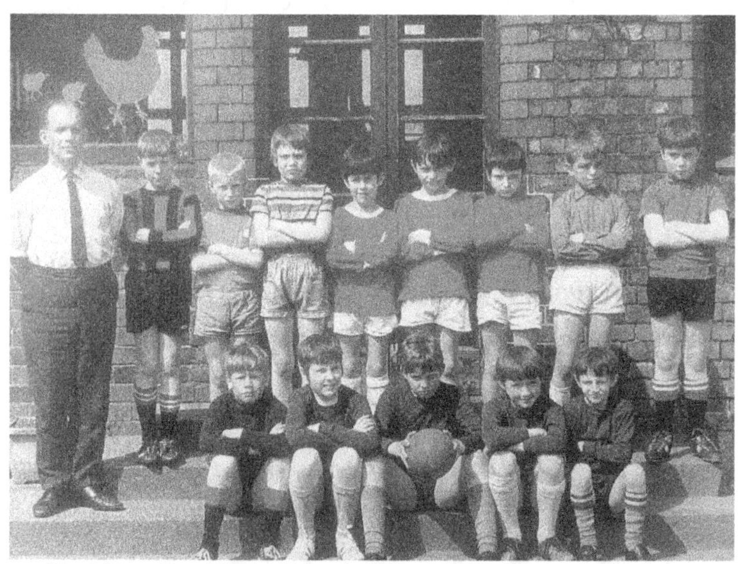

Blackfriars Road Junior School, Salford, 1970. I'm on the back row, second from the right.

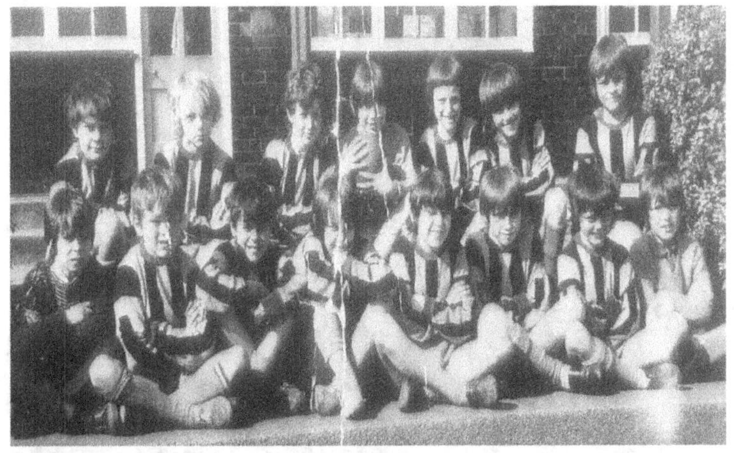

The Lower Kersal 1970s football team.

I don't ever recall playing a game for them but I suppose I must have. Oh, yeah, I scored a hat trick. You porky pier!

I never got a Buile Hill High team photo, though I'm pretty sure there must be one in existence. It eludes me, so instead I've included a class one from our house which was Lancaster.

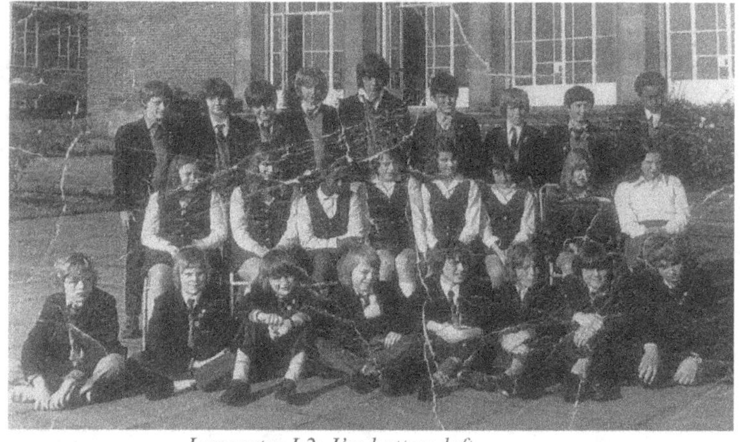

Lancaster L2: I'm bottom left.

When I ran the school 1500 metres, I was always the one who set the pace. I led the race till the death when was always pipped by the runners that hung on to my heels, Chris Golley and Mark Garrod.

And I think Simon Gore and the flash Andy 'Lightning' Washington, speedy bloody Gonzalez. When it came to the last lap, all those hanging on to my coat tails who had plenty in the tank would leave me in their wake. I didn't have the speed to sprint finish, I would be running on fumes and totally burnt out by that point.

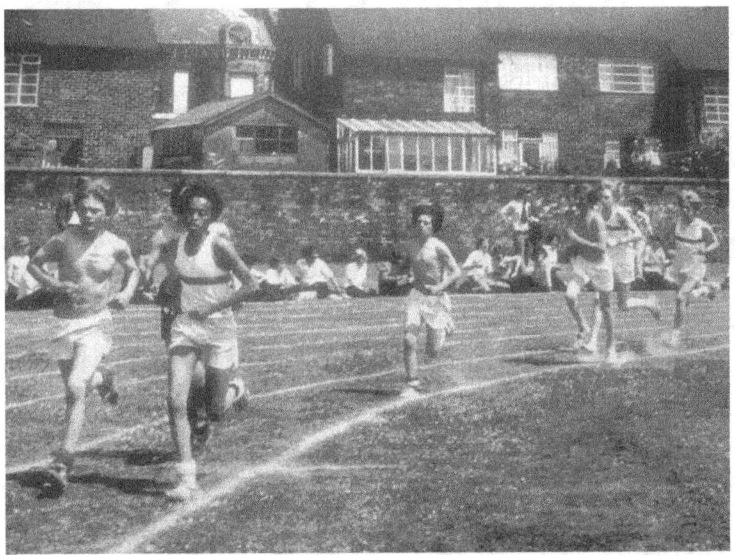

That's me far left setting the pace!

As for a six-pack, forget it. As hard as I tried in the gym, a physique like Rambo's eluded me. In truth, I found the gym boring. Give me a bike, a ball, or water any day all day.

Although I attended the gym quite frequently, looking back I would have been much better off channelling my energies in a different direction. Though, now, I'm realising why I couldn't work beyond my limits. I did the weights, the rowing machine and treadmill, and even though I wasn't fit, I did once try for the Gladiators, alongside Tony Darcy, Nelly and my brother Ian (Idge).

(Oh, my word, what was I thinking?)

I had forgotten till reminded recently that we tried for that show. The others were all a lot fitter than me, but only Nelly got to the next audition. In all honesty, that guy's a fitness freak. God only knows why I thought I had a chance, but eh, what the heck.

I think you had to do 800 metres in two minutes, climb to the top of a rope and something else. They didn't want contestants, they wanted Marines and SAS men. Poor Nelly did miss out though at the final hurdle. It just went to show the standard of contestant they were looking for.

As well as being a sporty type, I've never taken life easy. I've been a workaholic most of my life. I can't be doing with just chilling and I'm certainly not a lazy bugger. I pride myself on the fact that I've always been busy, busy, busy.

As a teenager I caddied for golfers over at Prestwich Golf Course. The actors who played Stan Ogden and Ken Barlow were the two golfers who used to pay the most money for a round (50p for four hours).

I also cleaned cars. I did Mr Birtle's van most Saturdays and was always gutted if he said "Not this week, son". I did gardens for the locals too.

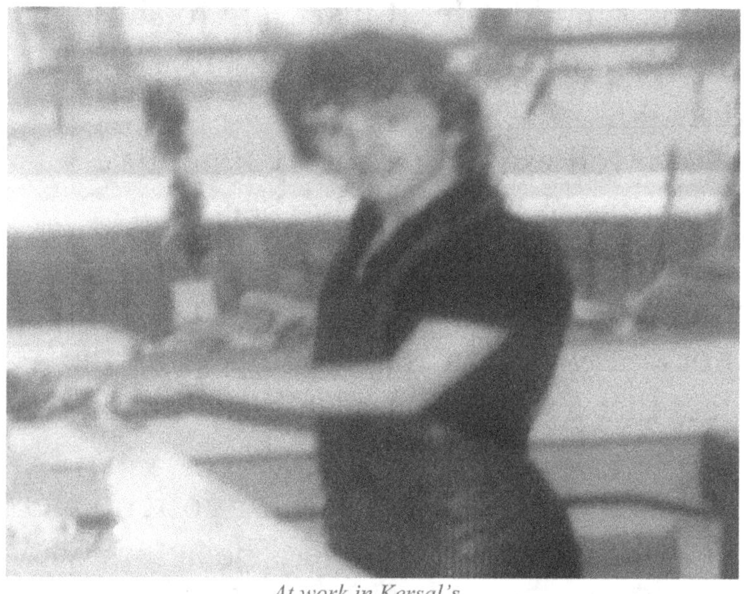

At work in Kersal's.

I even worked in Kersal Butcher's Shop and helped Saul with the Friday collections of the pools coupons. I also collected the empty pots at Lower Kersal Social Club.

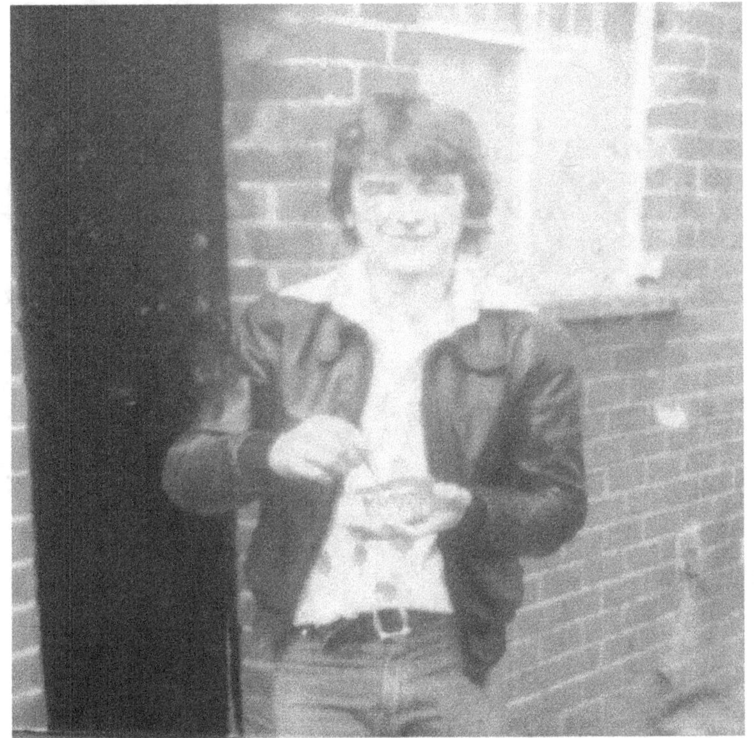

Me at the back of the butcher's shop.

Those working ethics have stayed with me throughout life. Where most people have a trade, I can categorically tell you I have a handful. I am fortunate enough to say I can turn my hand to all sorts to earn a crust.

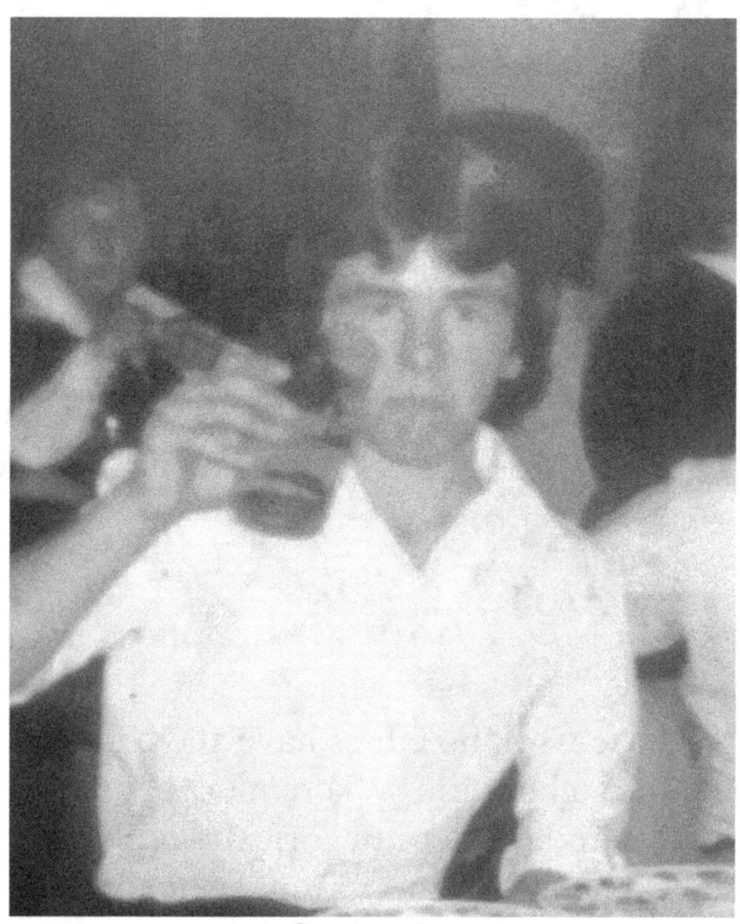

Downing a pint.

From my very first moment, my life wasn't in my own hands. What I mean is that when you're a baby or little child you are looked after by a parent or guardian almost 24 hours a day. This continues until such a time as you are old enough or capable enough to stand on your own two feet and able to function enough to make your own decisions.

This next photo came from a friend of my Aunty Mary's. I'm there in a white jumper, wearing a hat and with a balloon in my hand. I'm crying but have no idea who any of the other kids are, where it was taken, or whether I've bumped into, associated with, or even crossed paths with any of the kids in this photograph ever since. It is amazing how life rolls.

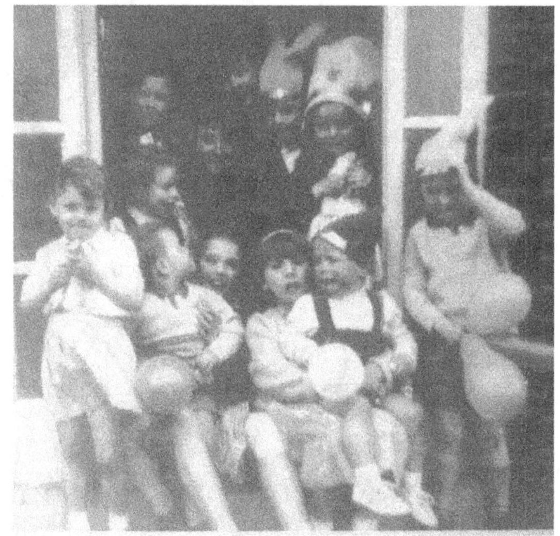

I'm the toddler with hat on, balloon in hand. I'm also crying!

The particular age of being responsible I'm not able to pinpoint, but I would probably put it at seven or eight years old. Maybe nine, as at that age I was able to look after myself walking three miles from Nantgwynant to Beddgellert. This was a country road with no real pavements and I came out unscathed. Granted, in 1969 there weren't as many cars on the road as there are today when it isn't safe to walk even a few hundred yards with ease.

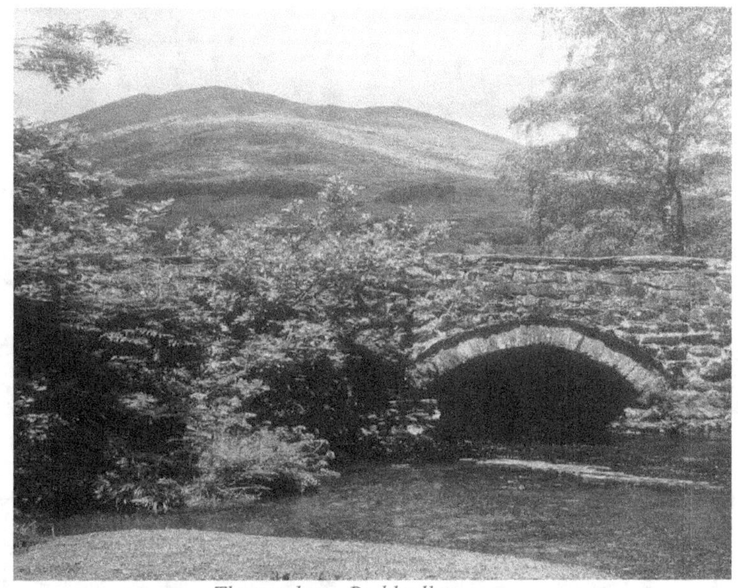

The road to... Beddgellert.

The road to Beddgellert from Nantgwynant where I stayed on many an occasion in the very late 1960s, the days of the Sergeant Pepper Beatles album.

The road would take me from this fantastic bridge going onwards and upwards past all the wonderful views that grace the Snowdonia National Park in North Wales.

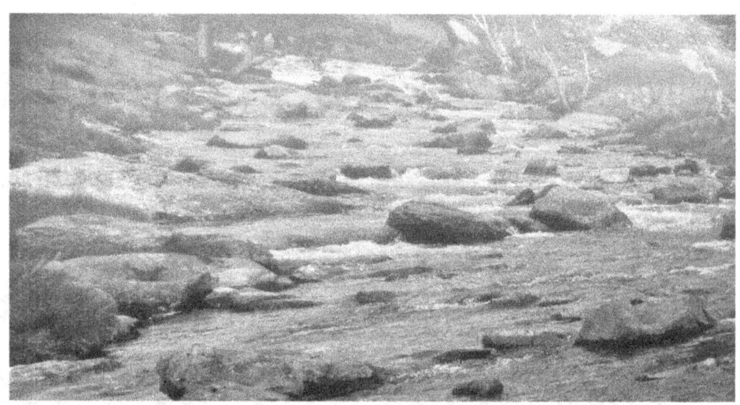

Along the road to Beddgellert.

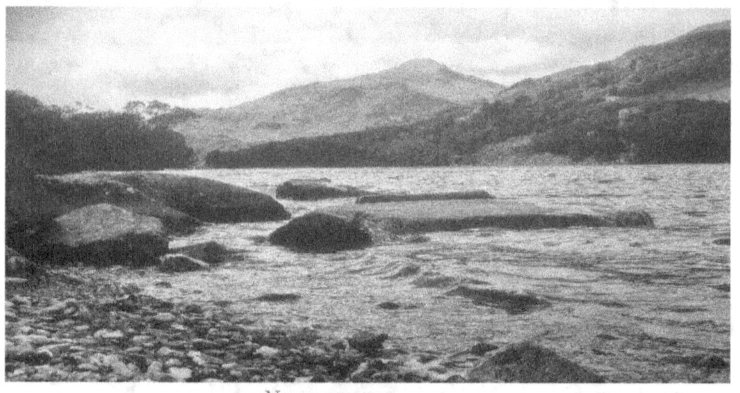

Nantgwynant.

I have such fantastic memories of swimming in those icy cold waters.

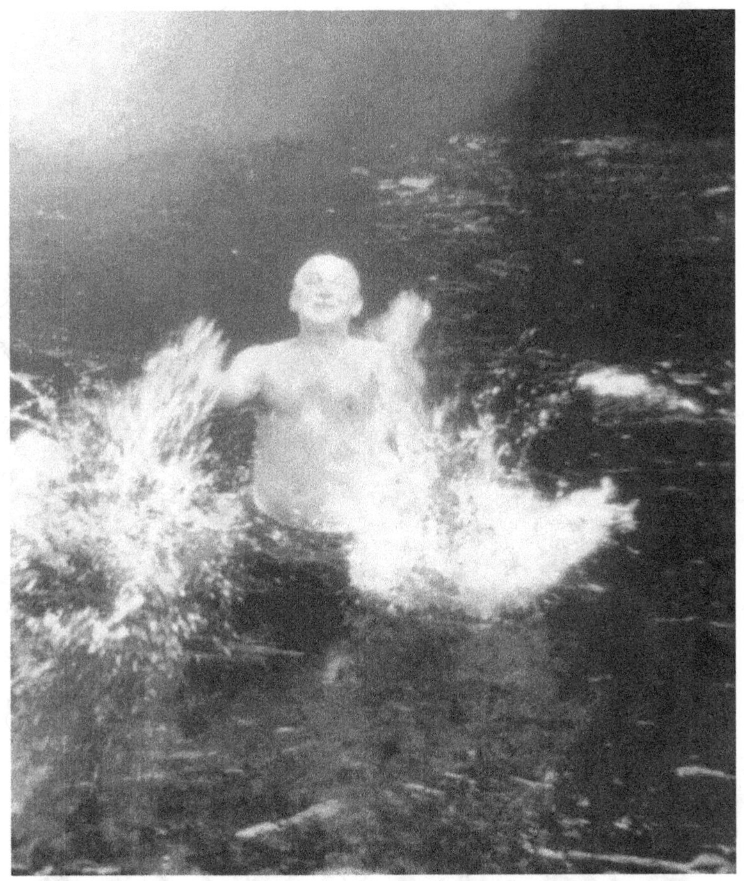

Guess who. Guess where.

And I still do it today!

My dad in his Austin - one of a few cars on the road, back in those days.

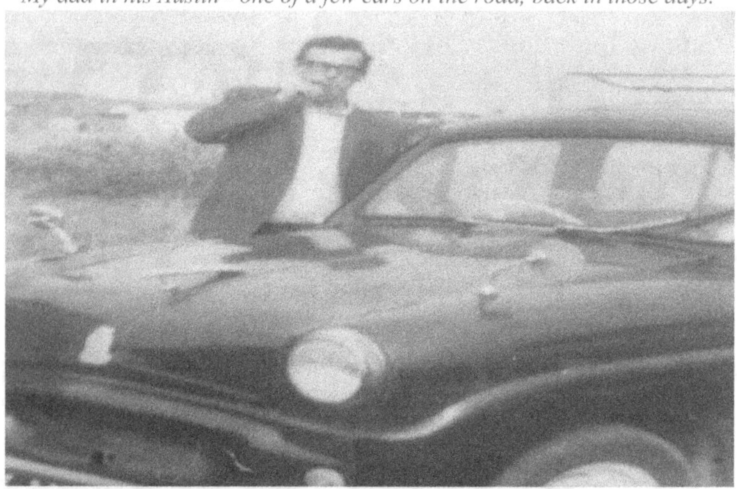

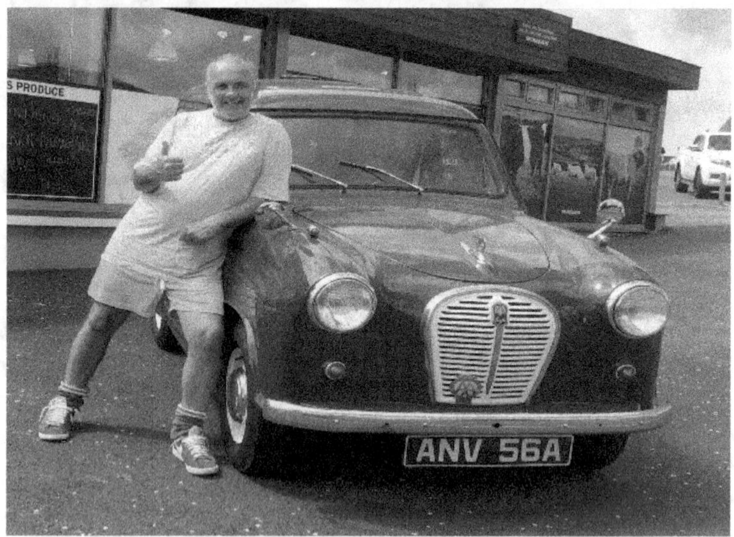

Me and an oldie car.

There may have been fewer cars on the road in them days but some of the cars from then are still on the road today.

Another of life's golden oldie vehicles was a Bedford van but I always called it the 'Campbell' when I saw one. Gordon Campbell's dad had two of them for years.

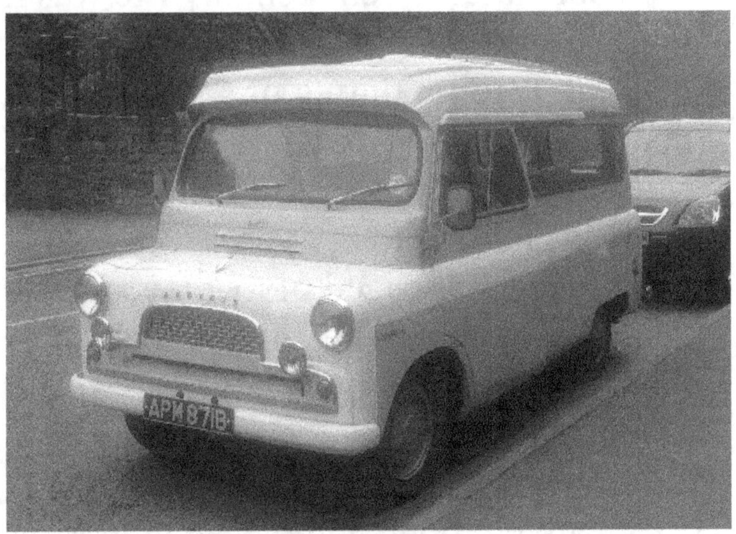
The Bedford Van

So, getting back to the point... It is 8am and I'm wheeled from my room to another just outside the theatre.

"Good morning, Mr Birkin. How are you?" said the polite nurse. "Now, we're just going to give you a little prick. 10, 9, 8, 7... I was gone from that moment on. My life was no longer in my own hands until I finally came round some nine or ten hours later. Even then, my life was not in my own hands. For the first time in my life, apart from fainting or gas at the dentist as an eight-year-old, I was put to sleep and thrust under the knife.

I was chatting to my very knowledgeable friend of many years, Mr Anthony Martin, who enlightened me to the fact that at that point we are basically as close as we are ever going to get to being (without actually being) dead.

We are cut open and placed onto a machine to keep us alive, whilst more work to keep us alive is completed. What happened in that theatre or who was doing what, I've no idea. For all I know, there could have been a doctor or nurse who'd had such a bad week that they may have had thoughts of "I don't like the look of him" and decided I wasn't coming round... Luckily, for me, that didn't happen. Yes, I know that sounds a little dramatic but, eh, things could have been worse. Strange things do happen, haha. So, I came round in the ICU department and, as my friend, Tony Wroe would say a few hours later, I was "back in the room". He said it constantly, may I add, the annoying bastard! I have to say that the time spent in the ICU department was definitely the worst time of my life. Three days morphined up to hell. Aarghhh.

The ironic thing is that most druggies love that feeling, apparently. All I can say is that they must be mental.

When I first came round, I still had the pipe in that went down my throat helping me to breathe, as my lungs had been deflated to make room for the surgeons to work on my Alan Wicker... ticker. OK. I mean heart. I was pre warned it would be there, and told not to panic. Nonetheless it didn't make things any easier, so out came the pipe and into my hand was put a morphine button. The nurse said to me, "Hi, Allan, I'm going to give you this button. If the pain becomes unbearable, press it."

What she didn't say was to take your finger off the button after you've given yourself the boost. Oh my God, I was gone. I was continually drifting in and out of consciousness. My finger was stuck to the button if I'm truthful. It was awful, and the very start of my nightmare seven or eight days. I was in hospital for a total of twelve days, but it was only in the last three or four, I felt OK and ready to head home to recoup, and make my attempts at a full recovery.

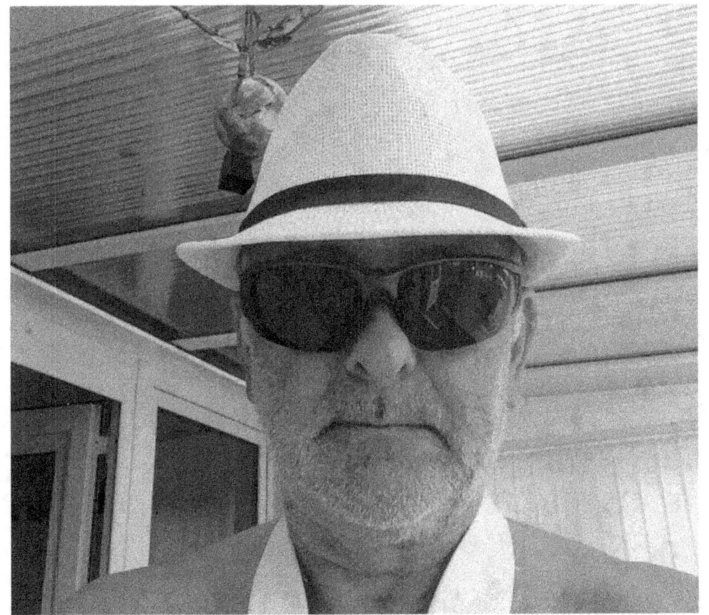

Cool dude!

5
DISCOVERING

SO, I ARRIVE AT MY unfortunate moment. I read an article that said instead of doing a 30-minute run on the treadmill you could replace it with an "as fast as you like two-minute sprint". That came from one of the fitness world's leading gurus. So, I had my target. It sounded good and, as I disliked the gym and boring treadmill anyway, I thought I'd give it a go. When I played five-a-side it was all short sprints and little runs so I had no trouble coping.

What's more, I enjoyed it far more than working out in the gym.

So, armed with my new-found knowledge I set off for the gym, and instead of my usual 30-minute jog on the treadmill, I burst the machine with the sole intention of doing the required two minutes. I didn't even reach a minute when I felt like Nelly the elephant and her entire family were sitting on my chest. That didn't feel good. It certainly forced me not only to stop, but also to never attempt it again. Steady and steady were obviously my set targets. After that little escapade, I sat down. I got my breath back and instead of thinking I'd just pushed myself that little bit too much, I realised that things weren't right and that something more sinister had just occurred.

I hesitated at first, but then common sense prevailed and I booked an appointment with the doctor. After getting past the person who thinks they're a top qualified nurse and doctor rolled into one (the receptionist) I almost hung up the phone. But, as they say, it's much better to be safe than sorry. Just as they also say, it's better to be late than never.

Getting an appointment at our doctors' surgery is not so different than with other surgeries. It is a mean feat in itself. Let me tell you, I've absolutely no idea why the women or people who work there actually work there. At times they are about as helpful as an ashtray on a motorbike. They rarely answer the phone and then they all think they are qualified as doctors. Their best line is "What's up with you?", like they can help, or are even qualified to offer advice. They know Jack Sugar about anything. In my opinion, they are just a bunch of brown-nosed nosey bastards, and then comes the best - We can fit you in three weeks on Tuesday. With sarcasm I say, "OK, I will get the hearse to stop off on its way. How's that sound, Miss Receptionist/Doctor/Nurse".

Seriously, you could die waiting for an appointment. You could actually be at death's door and they would still act like were very busy (if you don't mind). They are littered with awkwardness. I thought I'd actually attempt to beat their three-week wait and I told them I felt like I was having a heart attack. All of a sudden, as if by magic, the receptionist found me an appointment from her book of tricks. It was only two days away. Unbelievable.

I actually never gave it all a second thought until I was in the doctor's room Number Five. She was a young lady probably just out of university, she put on the stethoscope and did her routine. "Little coughs," she said, repeated her routine, then said "I'll just go and get Doctor Picaro, a more experienced GP". Whooo, I didn't like the sound of that. Off she popped, and I thought, "Oh shit, there's going to be more to this than meets the eye."

Going to the doctors has never been a problem for me. It is the dentist I hate. I tended to steer well clear and avoid as much as possible. But, looking at my lack of teeth, I'm beginning to regret not knowing the importance of looking after my corned beef. I have nightmares of the dentist, especially after as a youngster being taken to the three-storey one on Regent Road, being under the influence of gas, and having tooth after tooth out as a kid. Now, that was one scary Mary. Noooooooo!! The doctors though, was never a problem. So, in he comes. "Morning, Mr Birkin". "Morning, Doc". He picked up his stethoscope and with a wry smile he started looking giddy as hell at what he'd come across. It seemed this check-up was a little different and more exciting than the usual problem with stomach ache, cough or pissing too often.

It was as if he was about to be the first to discover a previously undiscovered gold mine with enough reserves to see out the whole planet. "Just cough," he said. I did. "Mmmm," he muttered, "that sounds like a leaky valve to me". For some strange reason he seemed to have this fascination with leaky valves. He proceeded to tell me of all the famous faces he knew of having endured the same condition.

Then he commented that he relished following up or keeping a close eye on their progress or demise. He recalled Arnold Schwartzenegger as one he's closely followed. Eee he was a proper giddy doctor at my expense.

I was starting to think that the short, sharp run in the gym was the catalyst for my present condition. Maybe, just maybe, if I hadn't done it, I wouldn't be with the doctor worrying my little green or yellow football socks off. You can't help thinking all sorts.

"So, what do you reckon, doc?" was me hoping he'd tell me it was all fine and "Pop your shirt on and piss off, just don't try that again". He responded with "Well, I can't be certain but I'm almost sure you have a leaky valve. We will have to send you to the hospital for tests. It's not mega-important but it's not something we can choose to ignore either".

Armed with that knowledge, I left the doctors and tried my best to ignore what I'd just learnt along with the fact that I'd be going to hospital for tests. The tests would be ages away, but let me tell you when you want time to drag it does exactly the opposite. Just as when you're a kid and holidays, birthdays and Christmas are looming and take forever to arrive. Sod's law, the four months to my hospital appointment went like a flick of a switch, but, as I'd heard a million times... the older you get, the faster time goes.

I got my first hospital appointment...

A LEAKY VALVE

So, it turns out that I was born with it, and could quite easily have died with it without ever discovering I had it.

Having a leaky valve basically means that your heart needs a little extra help to function properly. Had I been a laid-back type of person, it may well have lay undiscovered. But I'm not and I never have been. So, at 53 years old,

I discovered what had been lying in wait all these years.

I'd finally pushed my ticker that little bit too far and it screamed out for help.

When I looked back, I realised I'd actually come close to discovering that leaky valve on several occasions, even as far back as being 16 years old.

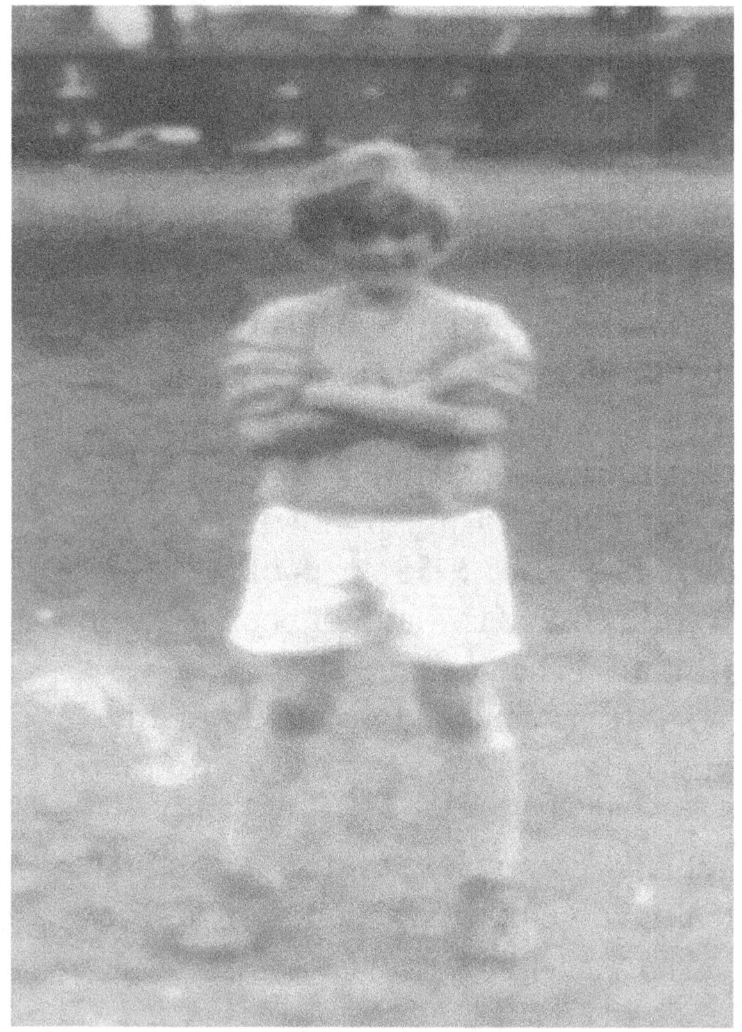

Me as a wannabe young footballer on Littleton Road Playing Fields.

<u>6</u>
HERE WE GO

S O, MY FIRST HOSPITAL appointment came at me like a shot. I hadn't mentioned it to anyone. Heart disease was pretty rife in our family from the mothers' side, the Coopers. Jimmy, Kenny and David have all had triple bypasses. Uncle Frank was not so lucky. One bump and he was gone. In fact, I was there throughout Uncle Kenny's to-ing and fro-ing to Wythenshawe Hospital, knowing secretly it was only a matter of time before I was going to be coming here myself for what would be my very own heart operation. Although I wasn't sure how far off my procedure was going to be.

I actually had that many appointments in the end for one thing or another I forgot where I started and ended. Haha, the old joke of his head being so far up his arse.

Anyway, my first appointments were at Hope Hospital and I've already got a complaint. The hospital parking and the fees they charge. Ridiculous. Don't even get me started on the biggest rip-off of all time, the TV and phone service. OMG, you need a second mortgage for both. Anyway, paying for parking is one of my biggest rants so that's a no no. I found two ideal places to park for free and they remained my first port of call on all my visits. You know (singing) "It's all about the bill, 'bout the bill, my baby".

So, I park up and walk in the hospital not really wanting people I know to know why I was there. But it seemed I couldn't turn a corner without seeing somebody I knew. I used to bump into Kev's dad almost every time I was there. I gave him so many excuses as to why I was there. Being there to see a mate seemed to be my most popular. He probably was shocked at how many poorly friends I had. Kev's dad worked there as a porter and just when you assume that hospital is such a big place you then realise it's not as big as you think. Every time I thought I'd go in a different way and go around a different corner, bang, there's good old Kev again.

At almost every appointment there's a procedure that usually starts off the same way. Blood pressure, pulse, weight and height, and the x-ray machine. So, I have all these tests to check on my condition and to position me correctly on the urgent list. One sentence that gave me a little ease of pressure was "We will call you back in about six months to see if it's any worse or if it's OK". Inside, I'm thinking "Please be OK" and anyway six months is ages away, or so I thought. Six months yet again went faster than a speeding bullet. Six months were like six days. Time waits for no man and passes in a flash when you don't want it to.

So, although I had this underlying heart problem, until I was told any different, I would just carry on as normal doing all the normal things I'd normally do. I was told my cholesterol was a little high in the November and heeded all their advice to lower it. I did try, but it's very difficult to change your eating habits of a lifetime. I cut down on biscuits, cakes and chocolate, with a little help and push from Yvette. I had let it drop a little, but I still kept trying. We've been eating porridge for breakfast instead of Frosties and have tried to steer clear of backstreet cafés and their big, fat, greasy fry-ups. So, I carried on riding my bike and playing football, especially my Friday night hour and half of six-a-side. I needed it and it was a great start to the weekend. Football has been a part of my life for over 40 years. I played for several teams over the years including a spell in this record-breaking pub team, The Star, from Liverpool Road in Eccles. I got it into the *Manchester Evening News* under the headline, "Amateur Team of the Week: Star Inn".

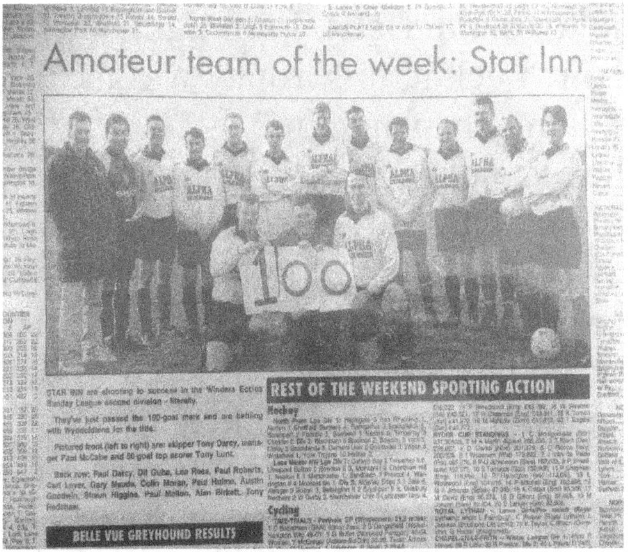

The Star team, Eccles. We scored over 100 goals in one season.

In all the seasons of playing football, like all other players, I have many a tale to tell. Some are of interest, and others just run of the mill. A few of interest spring to mind. The first is in all the years of playing, it wasn't until in my early 30s that I picked up my first winners' trophy playing five-a-side for The Jolly Carter in the Taylor Brothers' yearly competition. I actually cancelled a gig at the very, very, very last minute as we progressed from round to round. Haha. I felt tight but thought "Fuck it, this trophy will mean more to me than any gig".

Then I'm playing in a Saturday afternoon Salford League game for Park Wydyn. The referee was a complete dork and pissed me off from the word go. In the second half, he gave me a red card. My marching orders. I picked up the water bucket and raced back on the pitch to give him an early shower. I was stopped by all the other players, but I ended up in front of the FA committee in Chorlton. They banned me for 18 months across two seasons, and that was that the end of my eleven-a-side playing days.

But, on a lighter note. I'm proud to say I played football alongside a member of Manchester United's 1968 European Cup winning squad, Mr Jimmy Ryan, well in his 60s and still a class player.

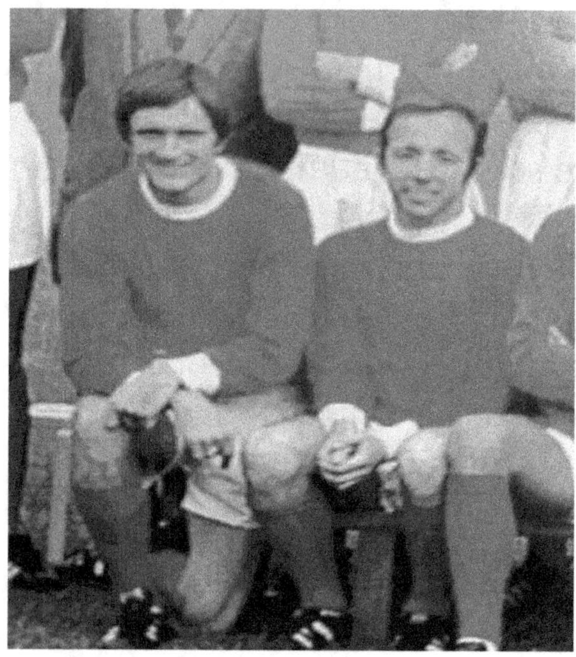

Jimmy Ryan with Nobby Stiles.

I also played alongside Martin Buchan, Scott McGarvey and Paul McGuinness, son of Wilf McGuinness and a massive claim to fame. As I played at The Cliff for the Manchester United's staff team, watching Sir Alex Ferguson score a goal then get substituted, only to be replaced by none other than yours truly.

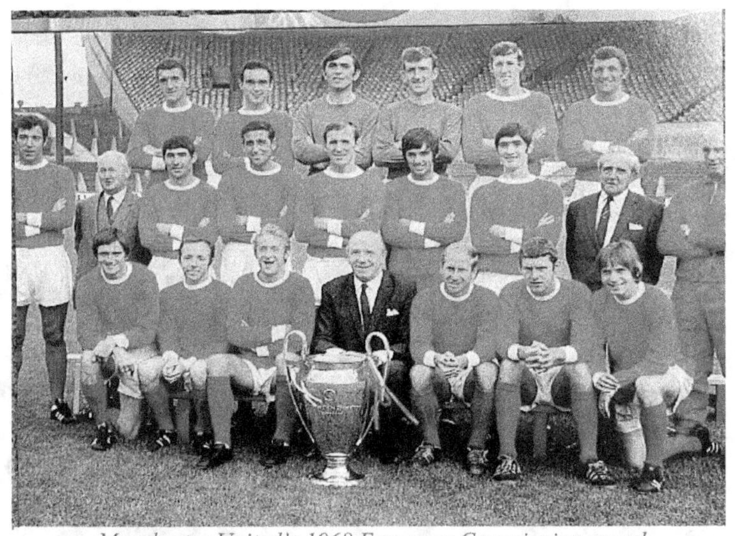

Manchester United's 1968 European Cup winning squad

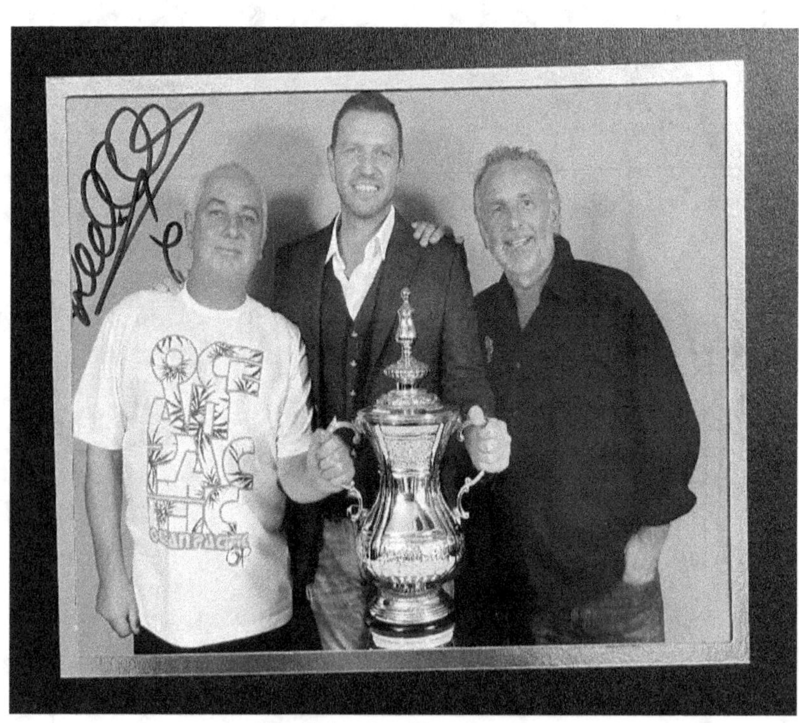

Ben Styles, Lee Sharpe and me.

I may have been 53, but I was still prepared on a Friday night shift. When I was playing, the first ten minutes were hard. Then I seemed to find a second wind and that spurred me on to the end. Thinking back now to a charity gig on stage at Cadishead, I was doing a tribute to the Bay City Rollers and struggling for breath. I couldn't get all the words out to the songs, and that gave me a bigger indication that all was not well. Thinking back now, that gig could quite easily have killed me. It could well have been "Bye Bye Baby" for real, and that would have been very ironic, haha.

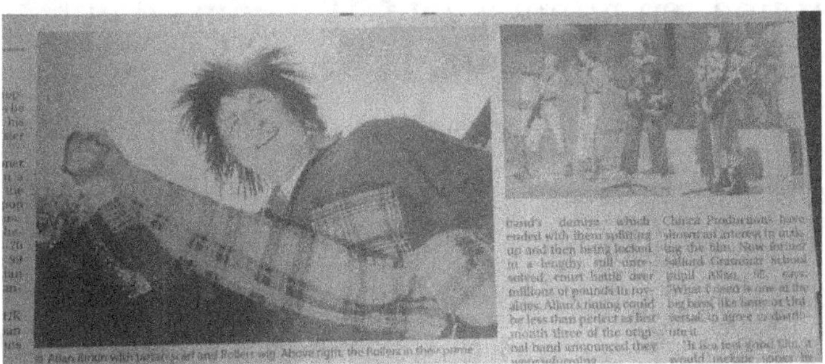

In the newspaper again. In tartan.

So, going back to the football, it was the sudden fast action movements that were causing the flow of blood and oxygen passing through my ticker to be thrown into chaos and not function in the correct manner. In my last game, and of all games I played there it would just happen to be the day where the camera system wasn't working (otherwise id have the exact moment on video), it was about 50 minutes into the game when I suddenly began to see stars before my eyes. I walked over to the boards that separated the pitches and I leant on them for support. The next thing, I was coming round ten minutes later. I'd conked out. All the lads were fantastic in putting me into the recovery position. They probably got a little giddy with the slapping of my face bit as I'm sure I felt a couple of left hooks coming in as I lay there unconscious and literally pissing my pants. They did call for help, but I came round, got up on my feet, and dusted myself down. The game was halted at that point anyway, so I drove myself home. I felt OK, but I realised that my footie days were well and truly over.

Although I had this underlying heart problem, until I was told any different, I would just carry on as normal doing all the normal things I'd normally do. I was told my cholesterol was sky high in the November and heeded all their advice to lower it! I did try, but it's very difficult to change your eating habits of a lifetime. I cut down on biscuits, cakes and chocolate with a little help and push from Yvette. I did let it drop a little, but I still kept trying. We've been eating porridge for breakfast instead of Frosties and tried to steer clear of back street greasy joe cafés and their big fat fry-ups. I carried on riding my bike with the lads, but the football was over. I couldn't risk that happening again. When I was back at the hospital I kept that little gem away from them, although I realised I really should have volunteered the information. However, in a different way on a treadmill test where they were looking for answers, I think they found it anyway. They noticed an activity that forced them to put a halt to the test. Perhaps I was getting near to the same point I'd arrived at when I keeled over at the football. I came away from the hospital that day with the knowledge my footie days were behind me and that it would just be the bike from then on. On the bike I could take it nice and easy.

I asked the consultants why they'd halted the treadmill test and, although they didn't tell me everything, I kind of figured from my fainting that I wasn't to play again or do any weightlifting, although I didn't need telling that twice. Anyway, stuff around the garden wasn't a problem but nothing too demanding. At this point I still hadn't told my family of my problem. Only the lads at football knew that I'd fainted, but I told them it was because I hadn't eaten. I remember playing footie with the grandkids, and Shani my eldest noticing I was puffing and panting. I made my excuses, but I felt it just wasn't time to let them in on my problem. I didn't want them to worry. No-one asked why I wasn't playing footie anymore which was good because I didn't have to tell them why. As we all know,

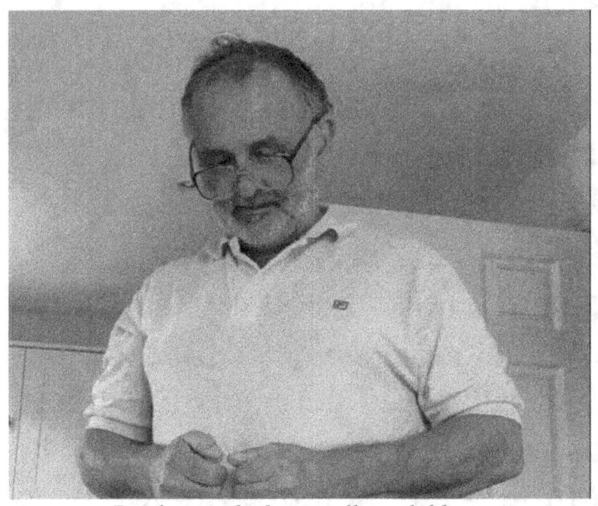

Pondering whether to tell my children.

there's no smoke without fire. I did have a close shave but still managed to avoid telling them. I was up in my friend Chris Littler's mother's loft when I fell through a skylight window that was hidden underneath some insulation. The glass sliced through my left leg and I had to go to hospital at Crumpsall to have it stitched up. The nurse did a fantastic job, but I almost had to tell them I was awaiting an heart operation when asked if I had any other problems, but I managed to avert it at the very last second.

As the summer was approaching, Yvette was hankering for a nice, relaxing break in the sun, but I was a little apprehensive about flying abroad. I didn't want to get caught out and have an episode in a foreign country and end up in hospital with a large hefty bill. Worse still, not be able to get back home. So, we went south to Cornwall instead. We had a great time, even though while we there we ended up and down what seemed like the white cliffs of Cornwall right near Land's End.

We were set to holiday in this country till some bastard decided to borrow our car without our permission and with our keys. I mean, I did leave them in the ignition with the engine running. I momentarily stepped out of the vehicle to inspect the contents of a skip. After all, it is my motto:

"One Man's Rubbish is Another Man's Gold".

7
THE SIGNS

S O, AS I AWAIT MY appointment with destiny I would like to go over a few pointers that I now see as possible signs of my impending heart problem. You could say it started as far back as 1977 when I was 16 years old. In search of an apprenticeship, I had an interview at Ward and Goldstones, the engineering factory on Fredrick Road in Salford. God knows why I went there. I couldn't ever have imagined being a grease monkey all day. Perhaps it was just a job, and back then I probably thought that any job would do. Needless to say, my heart problem, for once, worked in my favour. I didn't get offered the apprenticeship, and why? Maybe I wasn't keen enough or maybe it was due to the fact that I fainted at the interview haha! It's funny to laugh at that now.

Let me tell you, that story was all around school before I even got there the very next day. I put it down to the fact that I was suited and booted and my tie was on too tight. That was my excuse and I stuck with it.

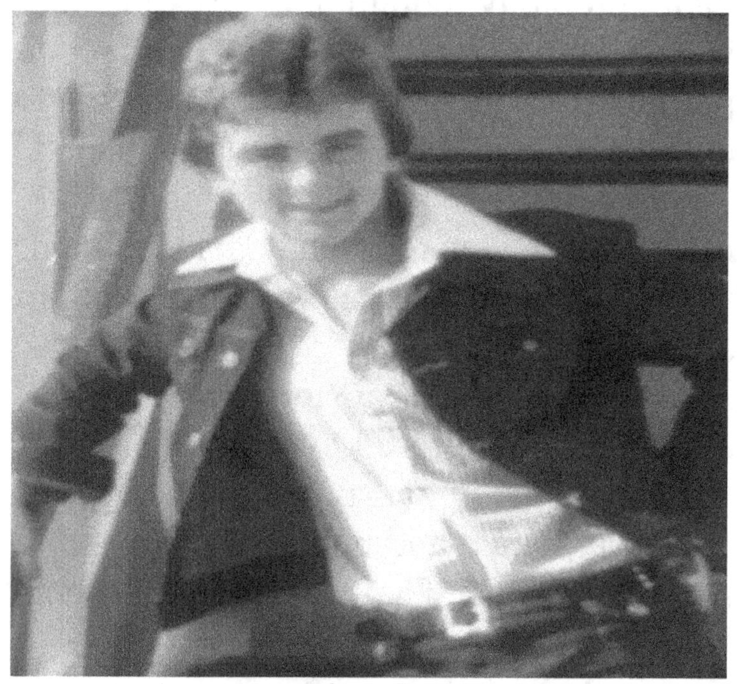

A young me on a ship to Germany on my own.

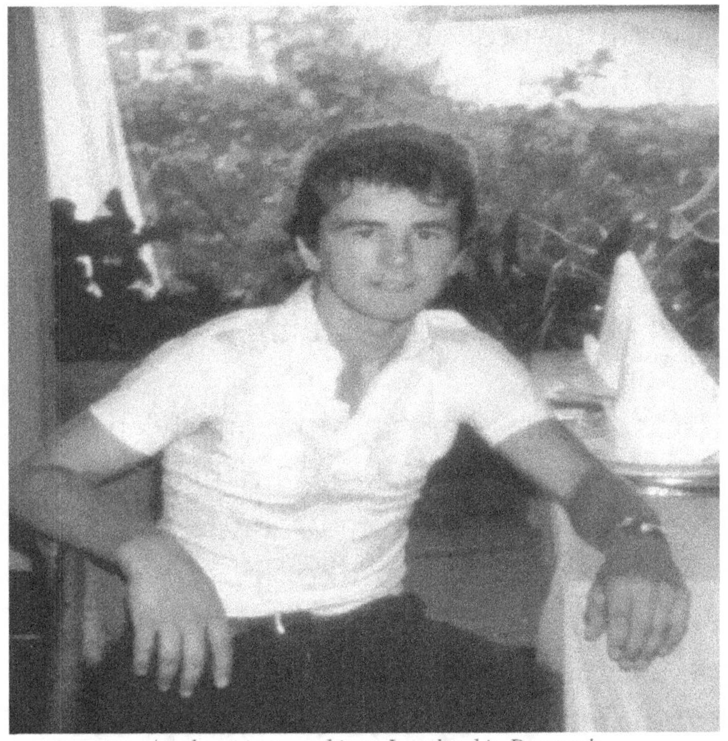

Another trip on a ship to Legoland in Denmark.

My second brush with the law of physics was at the latter end of 1987. I was playing five-a-side at the Eccles Recreation Centre one Friday night, from 6-7pm. Forty minutes in, a tackle from behind from no other than Tony Darcy. I soldiered on, but there was definitely something broken in my foot. By the time I got home it had swollen so badly I couldn't walk. I ended up calling an ambulance. The medic touched my ankle in just the right spot and bang, I was gone yet again. I can't say whether it was the pain or yet again something to do with my ticker.

One thing I can say now and I will put this down to the fact that my heart was not a fully functioning organ, was my lack of ability to run like Speedy Gonzalez. At a steady pace I was fine, but on a rapid boost, definitely not. For years I thought it was a lack of stamina, and now I feel that I was never able to boost and use excess stamina in times of need because of my underlying heart defect. As a kid, I found the fairground OK and the rides like the waltzers and bumper cars were easily manageable, but as I got into my twenties, I found those type of rides made me feel very light-headed.

My third and final fainting episode happened in 2006. After a long, hardworking day on very little food, I'd gone to North Manchester General Hospital to be with Ashley for her scan on her due baby. As she lay on the bed, getting ready to be examined, I felt very light-headed and ready to flake out. Ashley got off the bed and I immediately jumped onto it. I was out again. My third time. I came round pretty quickly and proceeded to eat some biscuits, thinking along the lines it was down to a lack of sugar. Thinking back now, it was obvious that my light-headedness and faints were due to my leaky valve, but at that point I didn't know I had one, meaning those incidents wouldn't ever be necessarily connected.

With those three incidents and my final fainting at football, I had a couple of light-headed moments that I now connect again to my valve. I was having breakfast in the café with Ashley, when, all of a sudden it appeared that we had just driven over a hill doing 150 mph, but we were static. I said to Ashley, "Did you just feel that then?" "No," she said. So, it was just me as a light headed wave passed right through me. I had one more of those light-headed moments as I was walking along the path at the side of our house. I sat down, closed my eyes and hoped for the best. The moment passed, and so... here we are...

<u>8</u>
ONWARDS
AND UPWARDS

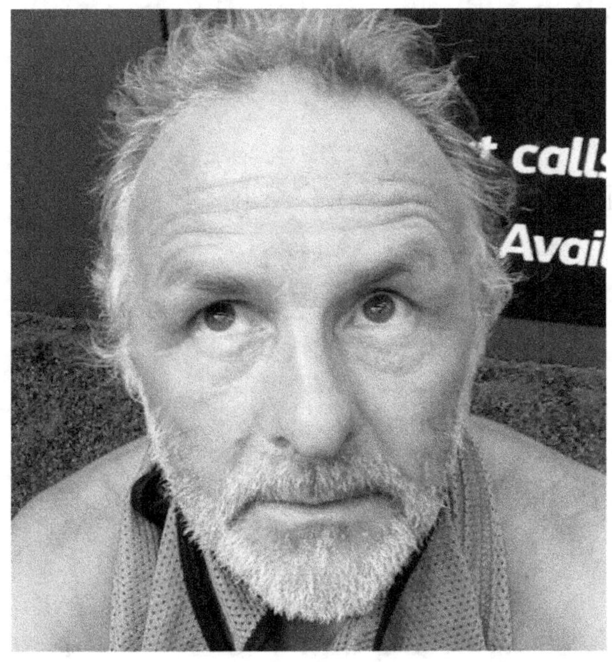

Me looking onwards and upwards.

I REALISE IN THIS DAY AND age that medicine and operations have come a long way. The progress they've made is fantastic, but it doesn't stop you from having strange thoughts and thinking "When I get put to sleep... it could be my last day".

Until the moment I'm back in the room.

Yes, I know it's a little dramatic, but, let me tell you, nobody knows what lies just around the corner. I'm pretty sure a lot of people who weren't so lucky felt just the same, but my only consolation is that I do have in my mind that when your number's up, it's up. Simples.

So, let's have a quick reiterate. I read an article, went to the gym, bust a gut, went to the doctor's, symptoms sussed, went for appointment after appointment, then got my date. Ooooh, scary.

So, I got my date for the operation after an initial first chat with Mr Carey who told me all about the procedure, what my choices were and what would happen afterwards. But, before the operation could go ahead there were a few last preliminaries to go through. First, there was a lung function test and a further chat with Mr Carey, the surgeon who was performing the operation, and a date for a further pre-op angiogram with a gentleman I nicknamed (in a good way), Doctor Frankenstein at Wigan hospital. Then, two days before I was due into Wythenshawe Hospital for my operation, I needed a final appointment with the hospital's Critical Care Unit.

The meeting with Mr Carey went well. He told me the reasons why the operation was necessary and what my choices were. There were two types of valve available to me – pig's bladder or mechanical valve. Choosing the mechanical valve meant being on Warfarin for the rest of my born naturals (days) so my mind was set on the bladder. It did change at the very last minute, you'll read a little later.

I was told that, although I had a date, if they had a cancellation, they may ring me at a moment's notice to drop everything and come in. I said, "Alright," but let me tell you there wasn't a chance I was going to take them up on that offer. I needed to be psyched up for this operation and I had things to do and put in place should anything go wrong. I was also informed that if I had a cold or any form of virus, they too would cancel my date. It's a risky operation to open you up, even more so if there's a virus lurking. So, I went back to Wythenshawe Hospital for the lung function test. That was a lot of huffing and puffing but all necessary as part of the pre-op process, and then it was off to Wigan for an early morning meeting with, yes you guessed it, Doctor Frankenstein. I would like to add, had I not been prepared to walk at least a half a mile from my park-up spots to the appointment rooms, I'd have paid a small fortune in car parking fees. I'm calling the doctor, Frankenstein, but the guy was nice really. He possessed a fantastic sense of humour. His lines were probably well rehearsed, but to the first-time, untrained eye, he was funny. It was also time to let my children know, so I broke it to them light-heartedly. I knew they would be worried, but I reassured them it wasn't a major thing. Inside, I knew it was, but hey, I'm there. What else could I do?

So, Doctor Frankenstein was a guy who made light of everything. I don't know why I was worried about any of this procedure as it was all fine.

I'm undressed gowned-up and lying on the bed, when in he walks smiling and singing his head off.

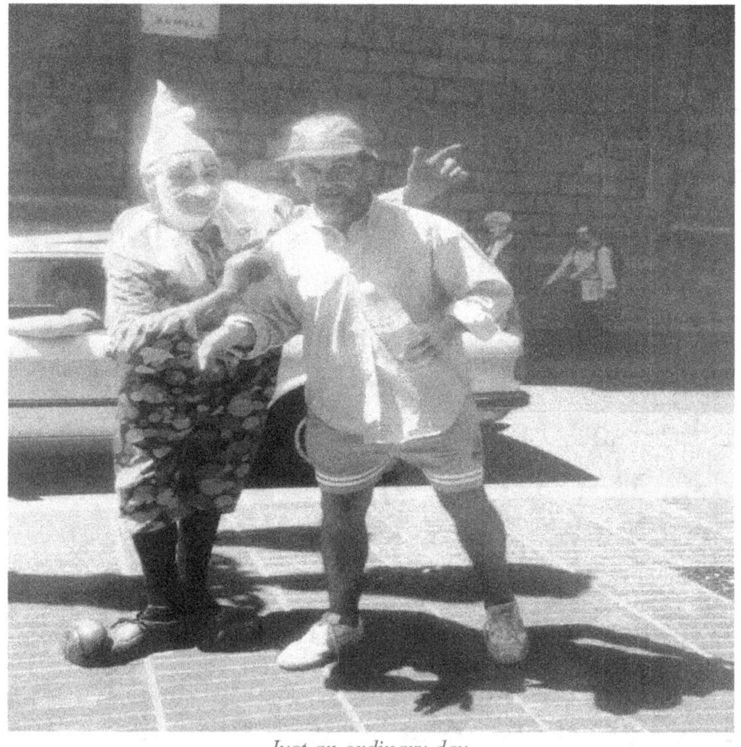

Just an ordinary day.

"Welcome to the Lottery of Life," he said. "You OK, Mr Birkin?" "Yes, OK, I'm fine." "Well, I'm just going to have another beer, then we'll get started," he said.

I couldn't do anything else but laugh.

When I was wheeled out of the room on a trolley and saw all the worried faces of the people waiting to go in next, I couldn't resist taking the doc's sense of humour. I said, "Oh my God, it's like Frankenstein's vault in there!" The pictures on people's faces were priceless.

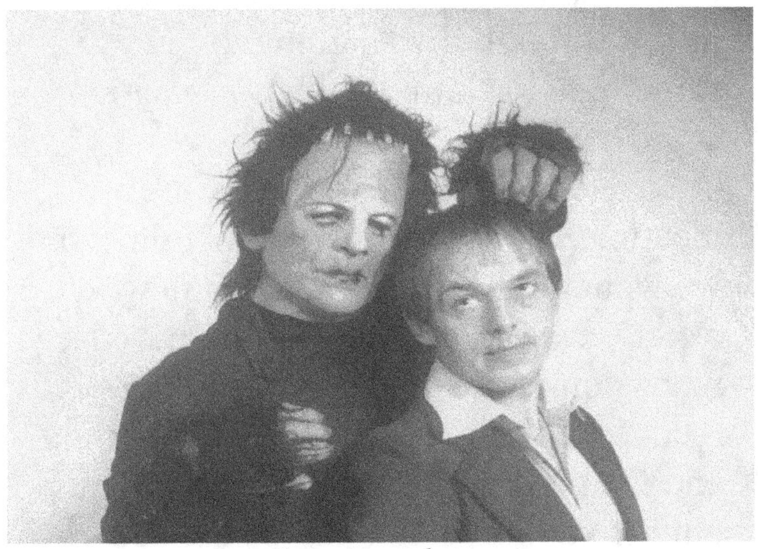

Not my pre-op doctor.

So that's all the pre-ops done. I'd written my will and spread out all the copies, basically cleared up all my loose ends, and my final appointment was booked for Friday at the Critical Care Unit, two days prior to me going in on the Sunday.

I could probably have gone in a little earlier, but I was waiting for the end of the footie season. Haha, yes, I know.

I also had in the back of my mind that if I pulled through, OK, I meant *when* I pulled through, I was going to give something back, in whichever way I could.

So, we went to the Critical Care meeting. It was the Friday lunchtime and we went on the bus so Yvette knew exactly what to do, bus- and route-wise when coming to visit me while I was in recovery. The meeting was enlightening and I came away quite positive, but on our arrival home that day's post had brought me a letter from the very same hospital, cancelling my appointment. A new date would be sent. The relief over me was noticeable. I was even smiling, haha! I know it was only delaying the inevitable, but to me, it was like a mini reprieve.

There were two more cancellations. One of them was almost certainly down to me for having a cold, but it gave me a chance to grab a few days in Cornwall. They also rang me one afternoon asking if I could come in the following day as there was a cancellation. I knew it was important to have this operation, but to me it wasn't a matter of life and death so I made my excuses. No way was I going in with a day's notice. I needed time to get my head around it. As I saw it, it was a do or die for me. I needed to psyche myself up. I got plenty of stick from family and friends saying my bottle had gone and that I was running scared. Kev, my son-in-law even joked, "Jesus! This is the longest goodbye ever!" I owe him for that one.

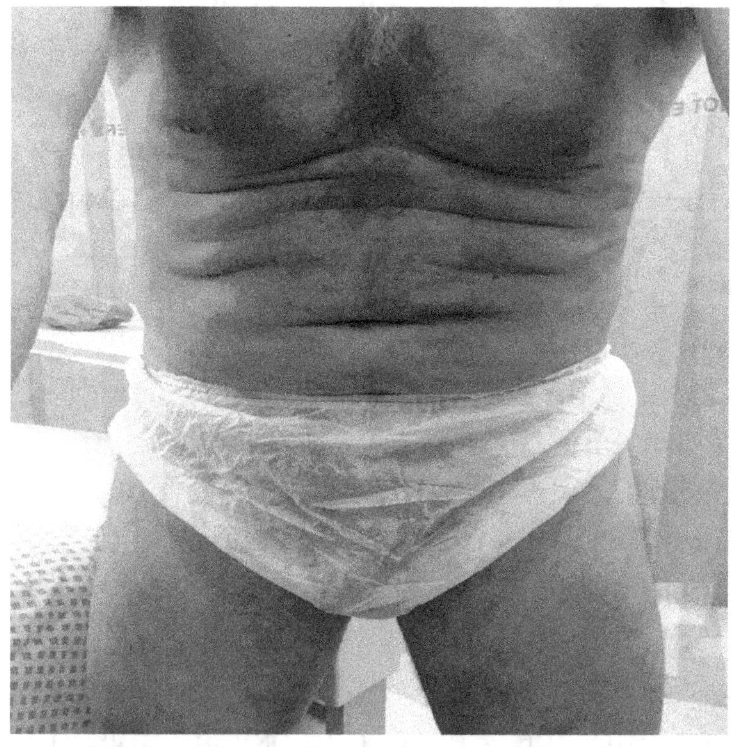

In my hospital undies. No, they're not exactly Calvin Klein.

9
IN WE GO

THE BIG DAY FINALLY arrived. Tony Darcy picked me and Yvette up at 12:30 and we arrived at the hospital for 1:00. I booked myself in and was given a bed in a room with three others. That was a good thing. The next few hours were what enabled me to change my mind on my course of treatment. My mind was made up that I was having the pig's bladder so I didn't have to remain on Warfarin blood thinners for the rest of my days, but as the afternoon progressed and chats were made to each of the three individuals that were sharing my room, my mind would make a dramatic change. There was one guy similar to me who was awaiting an operation. The other two had been done and were in recovery awaiting their departure. So, chap no 1 in the bed opposite to me had the bladder op, and if I was honest, he didn't look well. I didn't get much from him as he was more or less out of the game. The guy on the bed next to him was a gobshite full of the joys of spring, and very adamant he was going home that day. His departure was delayed due to his I and R levels not being exactly where they needed to be. But, oh, let me tell you he knew best, of course (not). He was still there the next morning, whinging about how he knew best.

By the way, that guy had received a mechanical valve, but with the mechanical valve your Warfarin levels have to be between certain numbers. You get a little blood reading from a hand-held machine which you can buy for about £300. The gobshite delighted in telling everyone he had already bought his, but experience now tells me it's not needed. I only go for readings every eight to ten weeks, so it's no big deal to make such a huge outlay. Then we came to the third guy and this was the one that really swayed my decision and made me change my mind as to which course of treatment I was going to undertake. This guy was coming in for a mechanical valve seven or eight years after having the bladder one first time in. Apparently, the bladder only lasts for between seven and ten years, whereas the mechanical could well go on till you stop. My mind was made up. I would have probably worn out the bladder in five years, so, mechanical it was. I had absolutely no intention of coming back in again, no way José.

Nothing to eat after 8:00 along with very little sleep meant I was wide awake from 5:30, and by 7:30 I was being wheeled to the patients' room. "Morning, Mr Birkin. How you feeling?" "Yes, I'm fine," I said quite nervously. Inside I was thinking "This is it. I either come back from this or this is my... Last Day".

"I'm just going to give you a little prick, Allan," said the nurse. 10, 9, 8, gone...

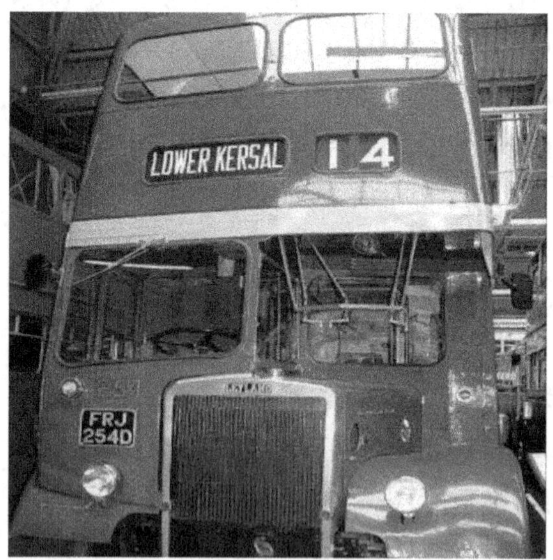

The last bus home... final journey.

<u>10</u>

ICU

*And, so begins the worst and
longest five days of my life*

THE OPERATION HAD GONE to plan and I was wheeled into ICU. It was about 5:00 or 6:00pm before I came round with the tube down my throat which was helping me to breathe. I was connected up to all sorts of machines and, as to be expected, riddled with pain. It is an amazing thing that opening up your body can actually render you pretty much next to useless. It certainly makes you appreciate just how fantastic a machine the human body is. The nurses in most hospitals usually do a 12-hour shift, so in the ICU department it seems they are your nurse and carer for all of your stay, but that's not the case. As one shift ends, your nurse disappears and almost instantly you have a new one in place, each one giving you the correct care and attention you need. Us patients not understanding that these nurses see this every day of the week. You do have a feeling that you want to reward each of them, with flowers and chocolates for the ladies and beer for the guys. They don't really want it, but you as a patient feel it's like giving them a tip as you would do a waitress in a restaurant.

Being in the ICU lasted just over 48 hrs which meant I had four nurses all doing their 12-hour shift, but those 48 hours seemed like 48 days to me. Time stands still. A minute's like an hour. An hour's like a day. It is a horrible thought. My first nurse was Tina, a nice lady with a very caring heart. There was a button placed in my hand. If the pain was too extreme to accept, I had to push the button. It was for morphine. What she didn't say or I didn't understand was that just one press would be sufficient. My finger was like a yoyo and I was morphined up to my eyeballs. I was about to endure both my first night in ICU and my worst. I couldn't sleep and time was standing still. Then, at 4am, I thought I was a goner. My body felt like it was shrinking, my heart was racing, and my eyes were rolling like an old 60s TV set. I remember being surrounded by doctors and nurses and thinking to myself I was going to die and had no phone to tell anyone. I felt I was going to die alone. But. whatever they did worked a treat. They managed to slow down my racing heart and stabilise me, allowing me to grab a little kip.

My second day, Tuesday, saw me cared for by a male nurse, Lewis. He too was so professional, and knew exactly what I'd be feeling and going through. On this day I received visitors, even though they were the last thing I wanted, especially one Tony Wroe, the mad, mad blue. He brought me a whole host of goodies and, as I drifted in and out of consciousness, was very repetitive with the words "Back in the room".

No offence to any of my visitors. Thanks for coming, but please piss off. I was in no mood for anyone, not family, not friends. Lewis's shift ended, and my third nurse appeared. Little Rosie, bless her. I was convinced she tried to kill me, by accident of course. I think she changed my meds and I overheard another nurse saying "Why have you done that?" I know, I know, I was just hallucinating, yet again.

Ashley did turn up to visit this day but I was in no mood. It's very difficult to explain, but it did teach me one thing. When people are in hospital, although it's a long day and very boring and repetitive, you still don't want visitors time and time again.

(I've recently been ill with a virus while I'm actually putting this book together. On the second and third day, it reminded me so much of my hospital visit that I smelt danger and dragged myself out of bed and drove off to A and E. It was a good job I did as my temperature was sky-high, my pulse was irregular and my ticker was racing which was stopping me from sleeping and making the clock slow down almost to a dead stop. Thanks to all at Hope Hospital five hours later, I was on my way home.) I survived Rosie's murder attempt, to be cared for on my third day by my fourth nurse, Joyce. She had the patience of a saint, that girl. She was tasked with getting me to do a number two. Under normal circumstances, that's not a problem to me, but this was a little different. I'd been diced and sliced and my torso was in shock! I did eventually reach Everest but not before to-ing and fro-ing six times. Wednesday tea time I left ICU. Those beds are few and far between and are always needed for the next patients. As I saw it, I was dumped on a ward. When I say dumped, I mean dumped. I was put on a chair next to a bed and was meant to cabbage there until the nurses looking after everybody else in there had done their bit and could turn their attentions to me. It honestly felt like hours and I felt like shite. I certainly was in no mood to be sociable or talkative to anyone. I made a couple of calls and cancelled all visitors for Thursday and Friday.

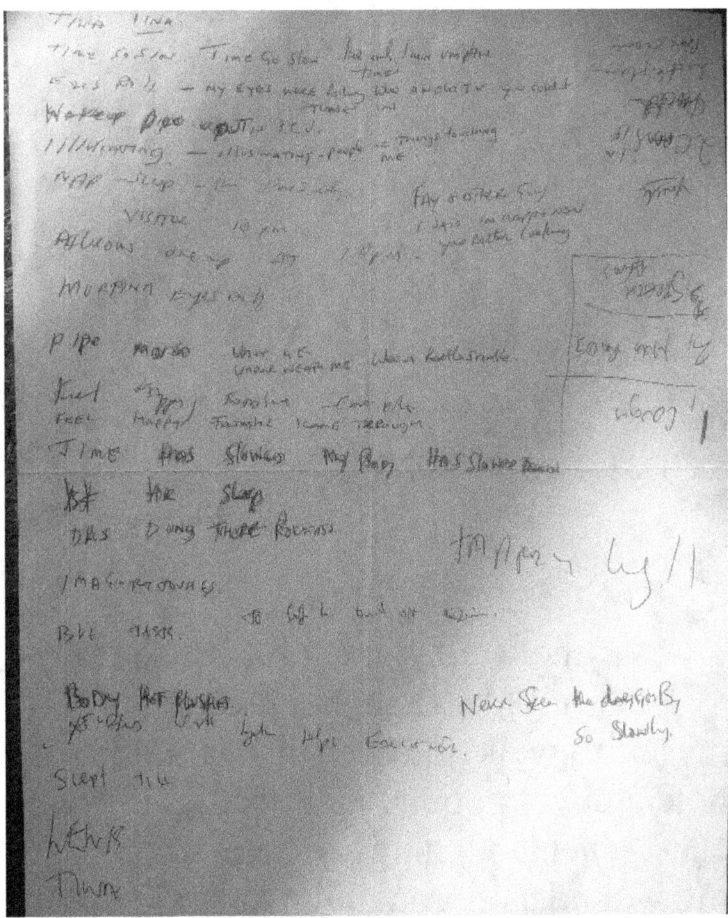

The quality of my writing in hospital. Aaarghhh.

11
RECOVERY

S O, MY FIRST TWO DAYS IN the ward were not happy ones. I felt like shite and had to push myself to walk and breathe again. I had to hold a towel in both hands across my chest when coughing so as not to damage my wound as I brought up the phlegm. I had a small plastic machine that I had to suck inwards that helped in the rebuilding process of my lungs that were deflated to give room to the surgeons who'd been working on my heart.

There was a gentleman on hand who was appointed the task of getting us to walk and climb the stairs. I have to say that guy possessed a fantastic sense of humour. I first met him at the Ticker Club meeting where he was on hand to do the speech. He was very engaging to all who were prepared to listen, and that carried on in his pursuit of helping his patients. A great guy. Top marks and ten out of ten.

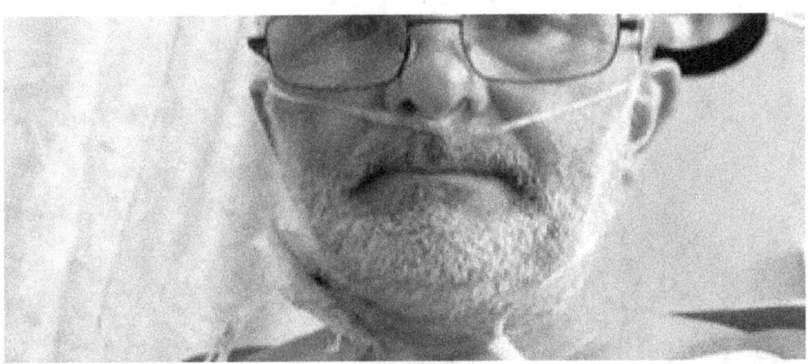

My very unhappy boat race.

I will say that being in hospital for what can seem like an eternity can have you listening to all sorts of peoples' moans and views. I will add that I didn't have any problems or complaints whatsoever, and remain ever so grateful for the chance to prolong my life. On those first two days back on the ward I had so much to do, and when you don't feel up to anything, it can all just drag along.

Because I was linked to several machines, getting to the lavatory was a job all in itself. I pissed all over myself on

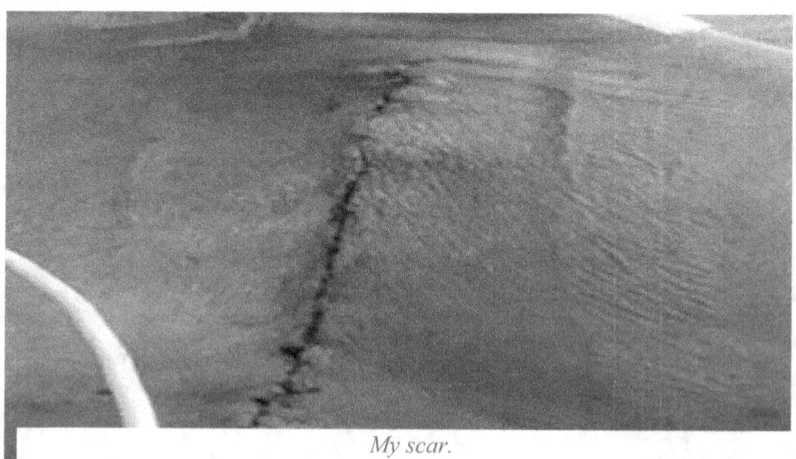

My scar.

more than one occasion and my bandages came off to reveal my scar.

By the Saturday morning, I began to drag myself upwards. I was up at 5am, brushed my teeth, had a wash and a nice cup of tea. On Saturday afternoon, Jack was allowed to go home. He was as happy as Larry, and I know they weren't his own, but he had fantastic teeth.

Here's a funny story about my ward-mate, Jack. As he was waiting to be seen by the doctors, he was impatiently sitting on the bed when a large group of doctors walked into the room. Jack sat upright to be seen, but they walked straight past him. I was in stitches as he shouted "Hey up. Listen to me!". The comic timing and delivery were second to none. He then got out of bed, grabbed his stuff and headed for the exit where he was immediately brought back by a nurse. Again, I was in stitches, with laughter as well as literally.

Eventually, he was seen and allowed to head home. Before he left, he was telling me about his old army day sergeant that he was desperate to find – a Mr Joe Fortune. When I left the hospital, I did visit Jack a couple of times and made inroads to find his friend. I almost got him a story in the *Manchester Evening News* and the interview was all set up, but Jack declined in the end. He didn't want to attract any publicity to himself. As Saturday was rolling towards Sunday, a guy in the next room who'd already been in a week and had still not been operated on, decided to open the Bury Conservative Club around his bed, much to the annoyance of all the other patients. At least 12 people were part of his Saturday night shenanigans. All that was missing was the bingo. On Saturday night I went to bed at 9pm, but was wide awake by 1am. I needed a wee and some of my cables had come loose, so the nurse brought me a bottle. She politely declined my invitation to hold it, but the male nurse did offer. "I'm fine," I said. One thing about a major operation is that it does make you emotional.

For some reason, I kept crying. I couldn't help it. For some reason, it would just happen and come upon me at any moment. There was nothing I could do to stop it except laugh along with it. On the Sunday, I felt much better and had

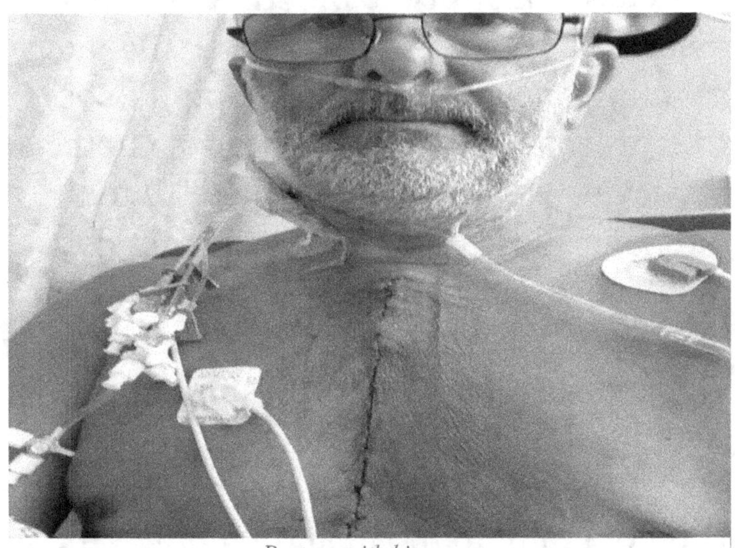

Post-op with big scar.

the two wires connected to my heart removed. I watched a little television and did a bit of writing. Ashley and Riley came to visit before heading back to the Isle of Wight, then, later in the day, our Tina and Joanne came with Tina's husband Steve. At the night time, Shani and Kev came and, as usual, Kev was on form trying to do the bedside Olympics with my lung machine. They gave me an extra injection to get my levels up then switched arms for the bloods. I didn't stop bleeding for almost half an hour! Monday morning arrived and I was hoping to be free of leads and possibly heading home if my levels were where they needed to be. I did have a loss of appetite. Apparently, the dishwasher in the kitchen was still broken and there were only so many times you can stand eating off plastic plates with plastic cutlery. It makes the food very unappetising. But it is what it is, and I'm not going to moan about it after all.

It's a hospital and not a five-star, all-inclusive holiday with Thomson's, as some patients are under the impression it is. In the afternoon, I got my results. They weren't good so I had to stay in. I felt a little down about teatime, but Jack came in for his meds and that brought a wry smile to my face. The guy from Wigan came in too, and he also looked a little peachy. Lewis, the male nurse from ICU, was married to a doctor who I met while I was in the ICU. She came onto the ward and I recognised her straightaway. She came in and sat on my bed telling me what operation she was going to do! I shit myself and then she realised she had the wrong patient! Phew, that was a relief. I was ready for a shower and a change of clothes.

On the Tuesday I was up at 5am, I'd washed, brushed my teeth, had a cuppa and was sitting in the TV room watching a programme where a guy and his wife were selling their house in Marsden. I was absolutely sure it was the moaning old guy who bought a house four-up from mine.

My appetite was back a little. I had two Weetabix, had my meds and spoke on the phone to Yvette, Ashley and Shani. Then it was time for my bloods. Fingers crossed that my A and R levels would reach their targets. One of the nurses I'd met on my second day in the ward was a very posh young lady called Fay. I think she was from Wales and she was the absolute double of Liz Fraser from the early *Carry On* films. She made a re-appearance this day which made me feel a little better as I got the results of my bloods. You've guessed it. I was going to find out what life was like in this hospital for a second Wednesday. Haha. What will be will be.

Anyway, I should coco... John, in the bed opposite, who came in from

Todmorden in an air ambulance wasn't allowed home because they had no home care in place for his mother who he usually cared for), then the guy in the bed next to me who was due down for his operation at 1pm, only to be delayed till 3:30. Then, as 3:30 came and went, he got cancelled till the Friday. They gave him a choice to stay in or go home. All I can say is that his home must have been very uninviting because he chose to stay. It takes all kinds to make a world. He did go down on the Friday, and when I called in the following week for meds, apparently he'd had a slight complication. I never got into detail, just smiled sympathetically and left.

So, my tenth night, Tuesday, was spent watching TV, then I popped a sleeper. Fingers crossed I'd get a good night's sleep, which in hospital isn't easy to get. I had a little pray that Wednesday would be my leaving day.

Over the course of my ten days, I met a lot of people: nurses, doctors, carers, cleaners, janitors, brew ladies and gents. A few definitely deserve a mention.

The surgeon, Mr Carey, and all who worked around him. I've no idea who they were, nor will I probably ever know. The nurses, Tina, Lewis, Joyce and Rosie on the wards. The nurses, Vim, Karen, Riora, and the posh girl, Liz Fraser-lookalike, Fay, the male pony-tailed nurse called Daryl, the gay male nurse, Mike Brown - the happy-go-lucky funny man who represented the Ticker Club and helped well with the rehabilitation to walk again. Also, the countless others that all played their part. No matter how large or small their role was, thank you.

So, I get to Wednesday. As usual, I was up early for wash down, teeth brushed, a bit of breakfast and a cup of tea. I sat watching breakfast television, my bloods were taken and again it was fingers crossed that today would be the day. The TV room was where incoming patients were sent before their beds were ready. I feel like, over that week, I had an advisory role, telling people about my experience of the procedure and how things were going. I told the stories that many times I became a little bored and decided to spend that day awaiting results, keeping myself to myself.

When the results came in... you guessed it, I was going nowhere. Talk about a downer, I was on the floor. My friend, Tony Wroe was meant to be paying me a visit, but didn't show because he reckoned that he was awaiting my instructions. Typical blue moon. Comes to visit when I didn't want him to, then doesn't when I do. Haha. Sod's law.

Bed it was then, and another sleeper if you don't mind. Zzzzzzzzzz zzzzzzzzzz zzzzzzzzzzz.

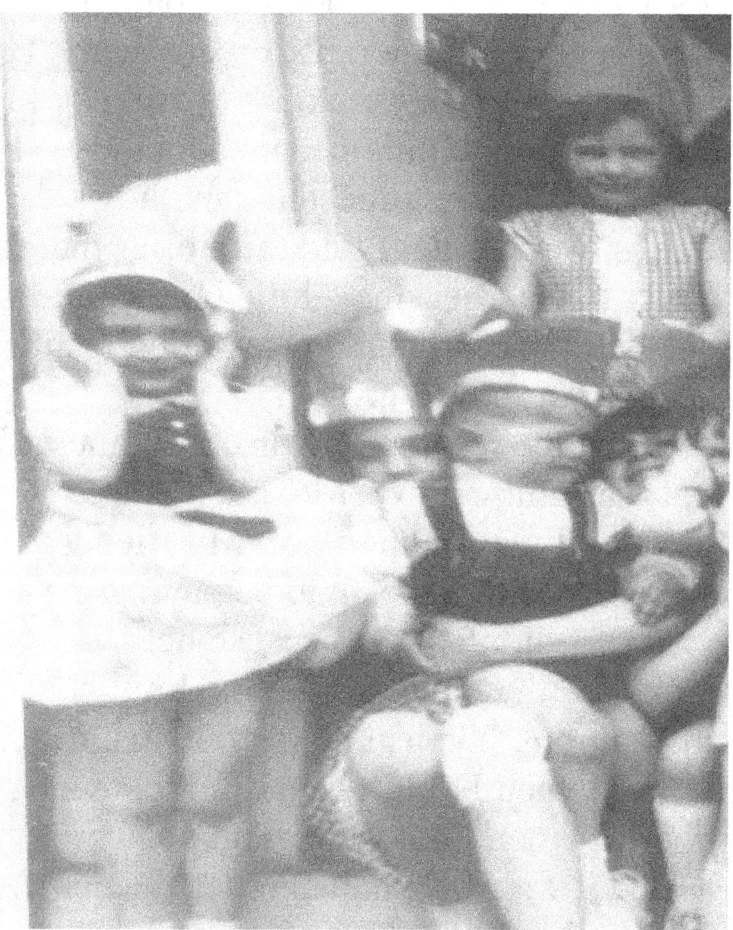

There are people who come into your life that you have no knowledge about. Nor do you ever see them again, then there are people who come into your life that you have no idea as to whether you have met them before or not!

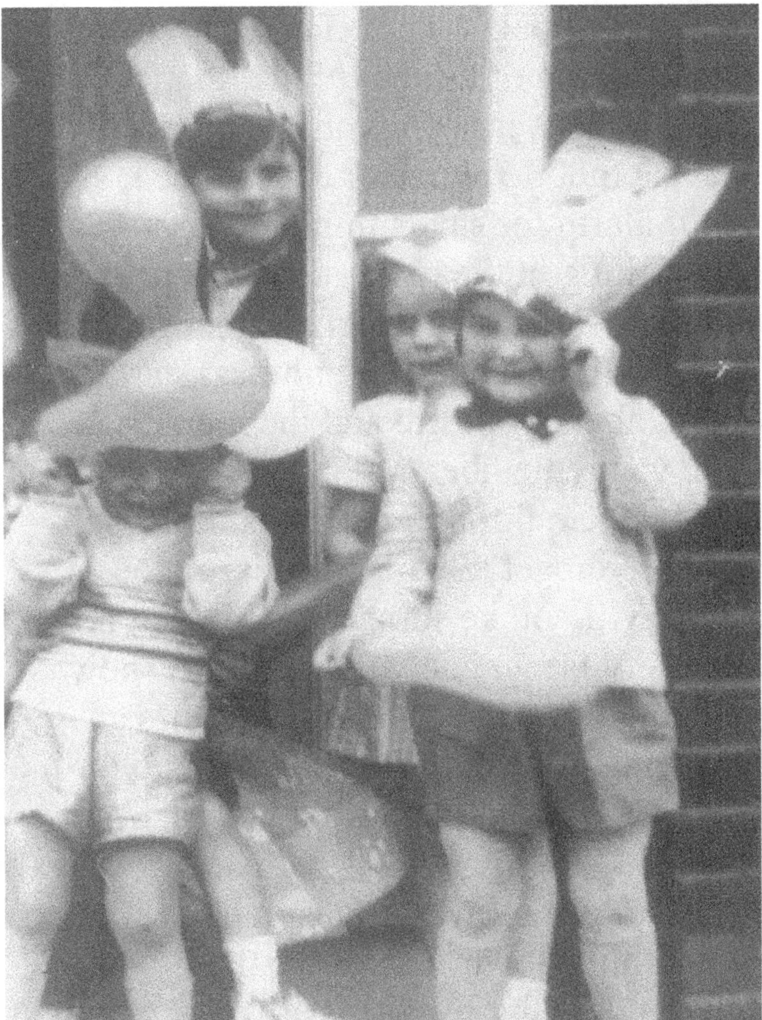

This picture proves my point. All I know is it was taken in Little Hulton about 1962/63 at a kid's party. I know of not one person in this photo nor do I know if I've bumped into any of them throughout my life. I find it all quite amazing.

Before I begin about Thursday, there are a couple of things I'd like to mention. The first is a task for your memory. If you have a mobile phone or alarm clock, set your alarm for seven minutes, turn off everything in the room to complete silence, sit back in the chair, then switch off. For the next seven minutes, start to think about your life and the memories you can remember starting at your very earliest. Go through the years. Let's see where you get to when the alarm goes off. Boy, will you be surprised, firstly at how not very far you get and, secondly, how much you will be able to recall. It's an amazing procedure and I beg you to try it, then try it again increasing your alarm time.

Also, when I was in hospital, I wrote something down. I can't for the life of me remember why I wrote it down or why is it so significant. I wrote 'FPV'. It stands for 'first person view'. Space flight. I've no idea why and I've tried my best to recall. Perhaps it will come back to me one day right out of the blue.

Thursday... Groundhog Day. Up early, showered, brushed teeth, cup of char and some cereal. I even had a few grapes, went to the television room, did a little bit of writing, took take my meds, had my bloods done and patiently sat and waited. I did forget to tell you that on the Tuesday I had to go down for a chest x-ray. I bumped into an old friend and emotion took over again as I explained what I'd been through. Typical that just like when I was having all my appointments and I was forever bumping into Kev's dad, haha!

So, the nurse caught me and I got the old finger prick.

I was praying for a 1.7. One good thing was that I got to lose the machine I'd been strapped to for a whole week. I felt like Tom Hanks with the football in that film

Castaway. That machine had been by my side for a week. It watched me shower, wee and eat. Guess what? I was definitely not sad to see it go and what ya know I never even gave it a name! Haha.

Yes, you guessed it. I didn't reach 1.7 so I had to have another night in. On the plus side, Shani and Kev brought Rome and Hermione and we all sat in the gardens. That was so nice. Shani even brought me some normal food (not complaining), I watched all the soaps then there was nothing left to do other than beddy bo byes and to cross my fingers for Friday.

Thank God, it was Friday...

So, I had to admit that I had a great sleep. I had such a good feeling about the day. I had my bloods done, waited for two or three hours... Tick, tock, tick, tock... Bingo! I made it, and was a free man. Even the doctors and nurses are celebrating with me, not that they were glad to see the back of me, but I think they too felt for me missing out day after day.

I made a call to my mate, Shrekky Boy, and packed up my bag for the fifth time. Dave from Oldham was in the bed next to me, was, yet again, two minutes from going into theatre when yet again, a transplant came in and he was cancelled at the eleventh hour. He was distraught and behind all my jubilation I really felt for him.

Lots of people I've known for years, and for many different reasons, are no longer with us. It makes me feel very privileged to be sat here writing this:

Rick Grantham, David Regan, David Harrison, Steve Corfield, Philip Lally, John Davenport, Dean Brennen, Alan Macintosh, John Denny, Paul and Steve Petricco and Carl Delaney. Bless them all. RIP.

But in true fashion of the circle of life we have new arrivals...

THIS IS HARRY

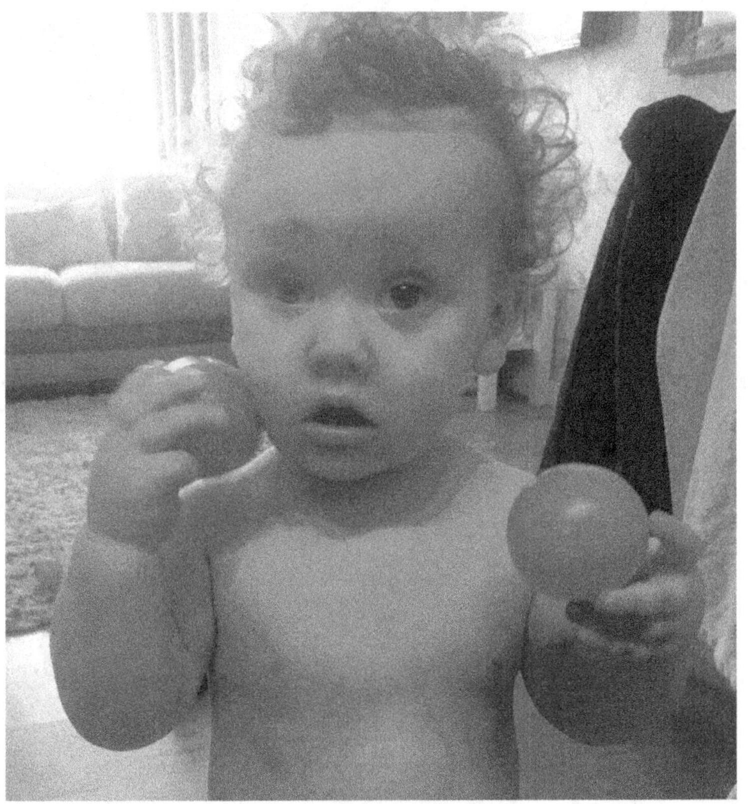

Harry, 13th November, 2016.

MAX

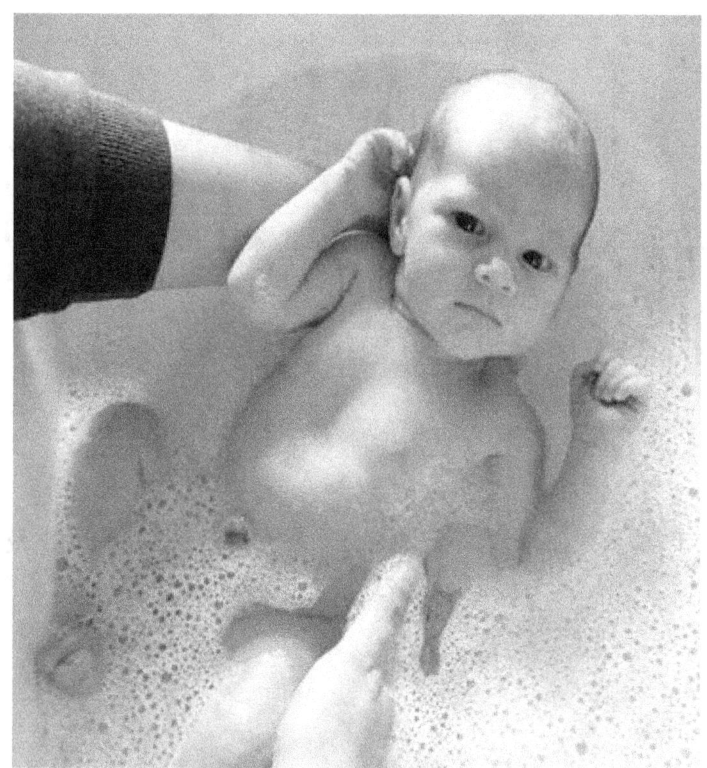

Max Paul Smith, 28th March, 2018.

AND, SOON TO BE WITH US...
OH, HANG ON, HE'S HERE!

ELLIOT

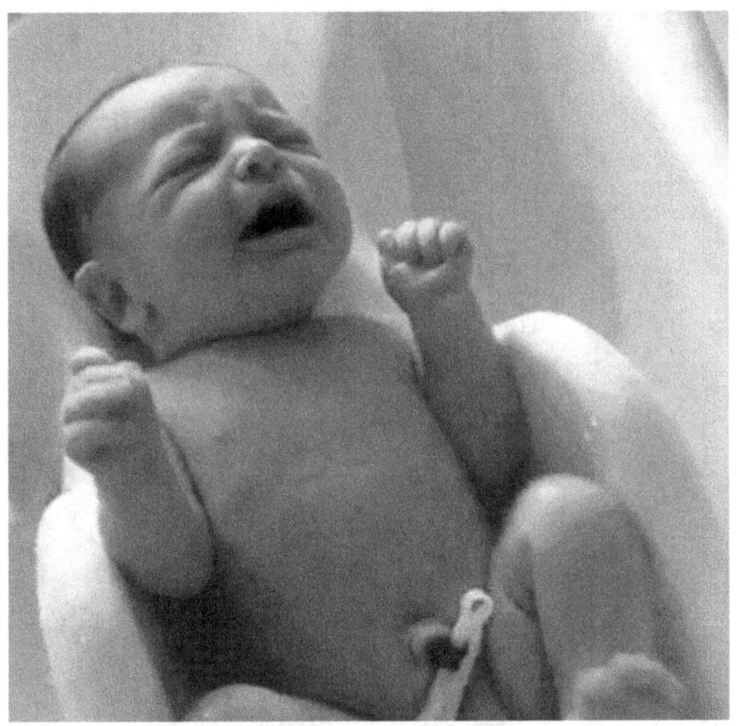

Elliot Albert Birkin, 18th May 2018.

12
I'M OUTTA HERE

SO, THE DOCS GAVE ME THE nod, my levels were up and I was a free man. I'd just have to come back on Monday for a check-up. As previously mentioned, I made a call to my friend, Shrekky Boy (Charlie Wynne) who was already at work as a taxi driver. Within 30 mins of the call, I was on the way home. It felt great, apart from the tenner he charged me haha.

I was still in a lot of pain, but that was nothing compared to the pain of carrying a machine around with me everywhere as I did in the hospital.

And so began the three months of rest and doing very little. That's the hardest bit for a man of my ethics.

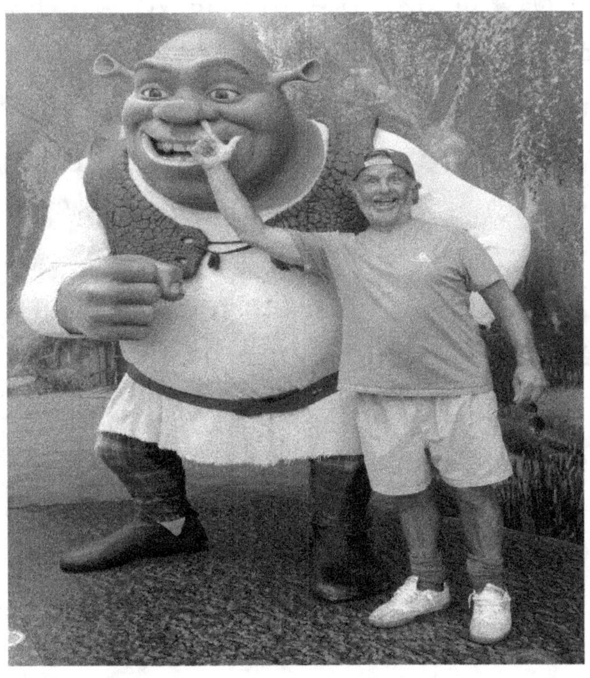

My taxi ride home, with none other than Shrekky Boy, Charlie Wynne.

The three months of complete rest were June, July and August. Getting up and down the stairs wasn't easy, nor was getting in and out of bed.

I did have a lot of things set up to do. A bit of writing, films to watch and lots of television were on my menu, and I was looked after by my princess, of course. In the August, I had to go back to the hospital where I was assessed and they changed some of my medication. By the September, I had an abundance of spare tablets.

In connection with the local authority, there was a special rehabilitation programme at Total Fitness Gym for heart operation recoverees. It was good and an education too. It was for eight weeks and at the end of it all they gave us a four-week gym pass, and swimming was included. Although I made use of the swimming and sauna, the gym still wasn't my thing. Boring, boring, boring.

I'd love nothing more than to get back to football, but I realise that not only am I not allowed but it just isn't going to happen. I'm still looking round for a group of walking footballers. It's a fairly new idea and concept and is probably right up my street. The principal is that it's for oldies and you don't run or have the physical contact that normal football requires. I know you've got to look forwards and not back, but I thought I'd have a little recap over my footballing history.

13
MY FOOTBALL HISTORY

THOUGH I CAN'T EXACTLY remember playing here, my football history started in this back yard at the back of our house down Lower Broughton, somewhere between the years of 1963 and 1970. By the time I was old enough, I made my one and only appearance for Blackfriars Road Junior School.

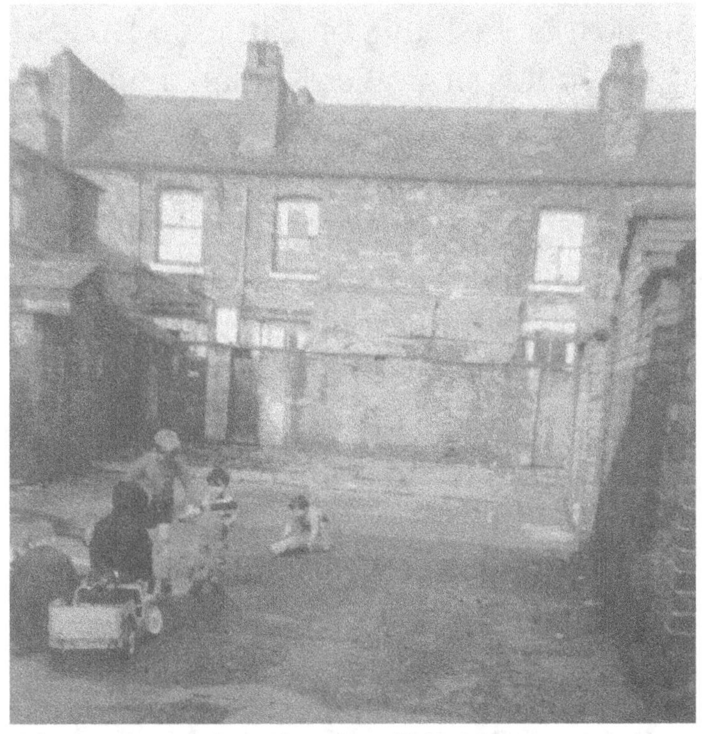

Behind our house in Lower Broughton. Where I first started playing football.

By the time I was old enough, I made my one and only appearance for Blackfriars Road Junior School. I was armed with no proper footie kit or boots, but loaded the winning goal in a 1-0 win against St Sebastian's on Littleton Road Playing Fields in Lower Kersal, a place I was soon to call home.

From there, my memory went blank, but evidence shows there was something I forgot. I have no memory of playing for Lower Kersal Junior School, but here I am as a fully-fledged member of the school team alongside the Skillen twins. I went to grammar school with them, went to college with them, and we rode our first motorbike together. I still communicate with Wayne, but Mark (God rest his soul) is no longer with us.

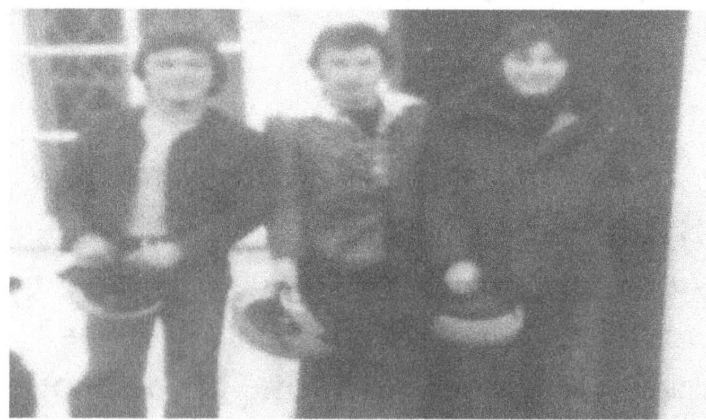

Me, Mark and Wayne Skillen.

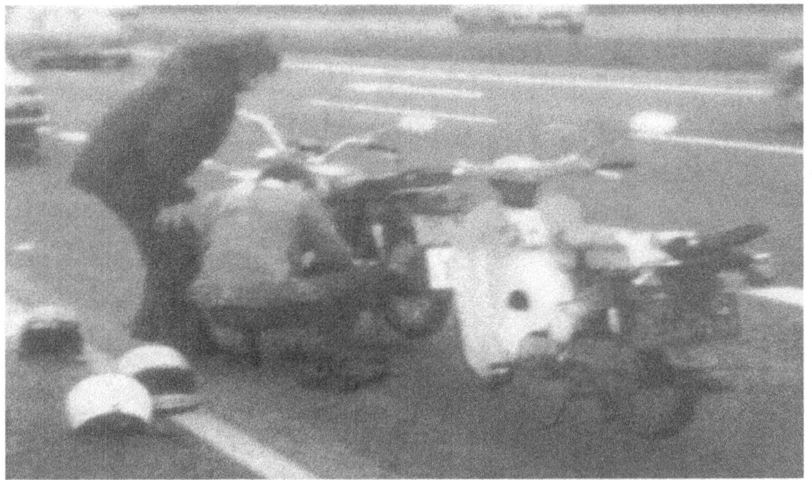

My first and only motorbike. I called it my Honda 50 with wings. I only bought it so I could learn to ride a bike for a part in Emmerdale Farm!

So, on to Salford Grammar School soon renamed Buile Hill High. There we had an A and B team. I was always a B team player. The A team was just too good to get into and had an abundance of gifted and natural players.

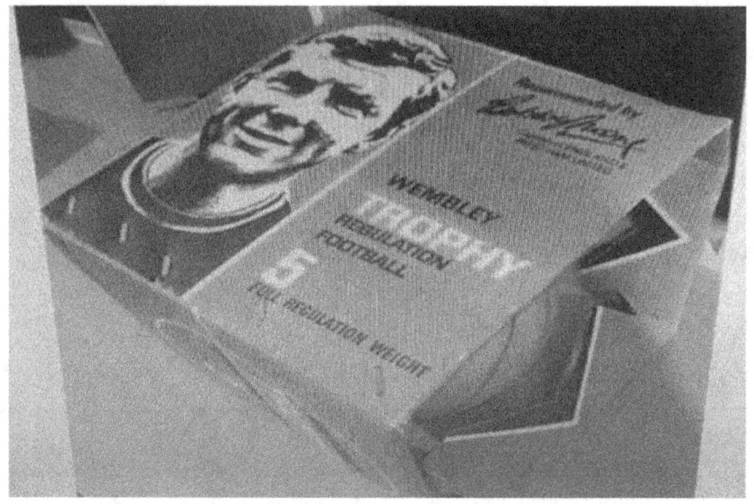

Our main football of the day – A Wembley Trophy ball.

Although, if memory serves me correctly, when the A team was full of injured players I manage to scrape in a couple of games. I think I even played in a cup final down at the Cliff area of Broughton. I really do need to research that one day and get to the bottom of it.

After school, football took a back seat until I once again got the bug and back into it through five-a-side and then 11-a-side on Saturday and Sunday. I played for the likes of the Jolly Carter pub based in

Winton, then Park Wyden and finally The Star, a public house on Liverpool Road, Eccles. This was all just for fun, of course, until I got banned for the best part of two years, for having a go at a monged-out referee, I had abused him throughout the game until he finally gave me the red card and sent me off. At that point I raced to the water bucket to instigate the Ice Bucket Challenge, years ahead of its time. I was apprehended by my team mates thus preventing the referee from receiving his early bath. Temper, temper, Mr Birkin.

When I played football, I feel I was fairly good at five-a-side and could hold my own, but when it came to eleven-a-side, I never had the stamina or lung capacity. Little did I realise that it was something to do with my ticker. Short bursts were fine, even doing the 1500 metres or cross country, but chasing that ball up and down the pitch measuring a few hundred metres to tackle, dribble and shoot was difficult.

Perhaps now I realise why it was all so difficult. Up until I was 53, I was playing six-a-side and eleven-a-side on an astroturf at Moston with Tony Wroe's team from Prestwich. If I'm honest, it was a struggle.

So back to the six-a-side. I did Tuesday nights at Ordsall Rec and at the JJB Fridays from 5 till 6. I loved the games, the good standard of players and plenty of banter and pitch battles. The first 15 minutes were always a struggle until I found my second wind. From then, it was onwards and upwards until the final whistle. Until that fateful Friday when, already armed with the knowledge I had a leaky valve, I started seeing stars before my eyes. I leant on the railings only to be brought round five or ten minutes later by the lads who thankfully put me in the recovery position and never giggled as I lay there pissing my shorts. Thank God for TENA pants haha. Basically, my footie days were over apart from playing once for over 55s. I had a very strenuous but funny game of beach football, which is well recommended, and I'm also looking into walking football. I did fall out of love with football during the 1980s.

<u>14</u>
SO MANY PEOPLE

URING MY THIRTEEN DAY stay, I met a lot of different people, be it doctors, nurses, carers, cleaners and other patients and their many visitors . The majority of people were nice. One chap I particularly warmed to, arrived in the bed next to me as I slept through the night.

He was 82-year-old Jack Males, but I kept calling him Ken, for some reason.

He was an ex-RAF man, pilot stroke mechanic and like myself a jack of all trades. He reminded me so much of myself.

Jack was in hospital because he had fallen while trying to cut conifers from a ladder. The guy was amazing.

I met him after our hospital stay and visited his amazing farm. I got to realise there was even more to the man than I could possibly imagine. He had a plane, a helicopter, a Rolls Royce... in fact, it's easier to tell you what he didn't have. He was such a nice chap and as much as I've tried to stay in touch, I got to realise that he's old and just wants to be left alone to enjoy his latter years.

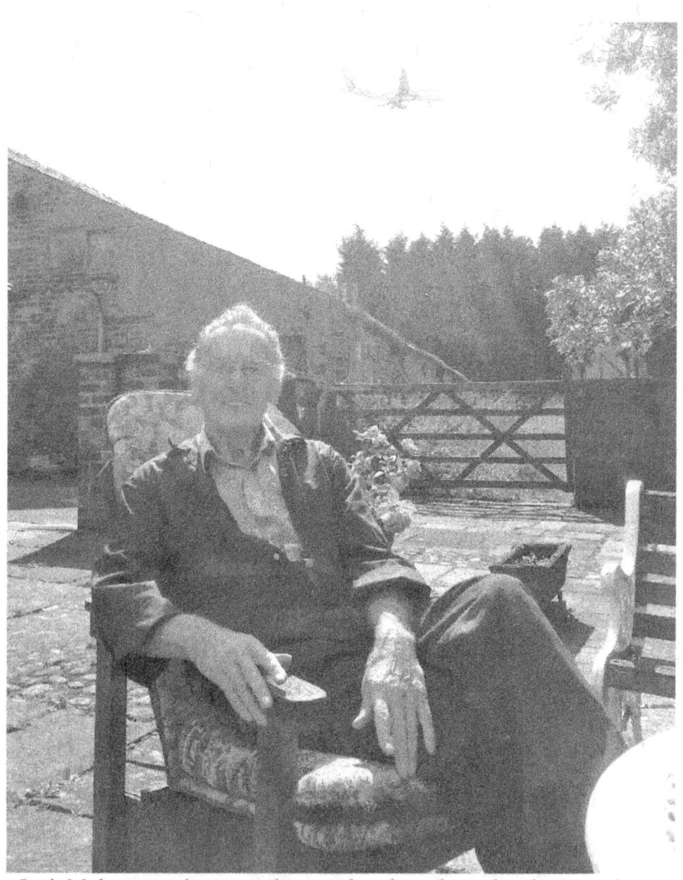

Jack Males sat relaxing in his garden directly under the Manchester airport flight path. Amazing man. Amazing place.

15
AFTERWARDS

SO, I'M WRITING THIS PART IN April 2018, almost three years since I had my operation. No, I don't feel like Superman, but then I wasn't ill before the operation. I just had a leaky valve that had ran on its own for a lot of years and decided it needed a little help.

I do feel blessed to still be here, but I will only be here as long as I will be. Like I've said before today, when it is your time and your number is up, that's it. Your number is up. There's no escaping that final destination, so while I'm here I will make the most of it all. I do have a lot of plans still to implement, but I know I don't have an eternity to implement them so I'll just keep going until I no longer can. I no longer play football, but I do ride my bike. I don't really do anything that makes me go a little dizzy. In the back of my mind, I'm always a little conscious about pushing my luck a little too far. On a final note, my mechanical valve I can hear ticking in the middle of the night like Big Ben does so over 32 million times a year. It is an amazing piece of equipment.

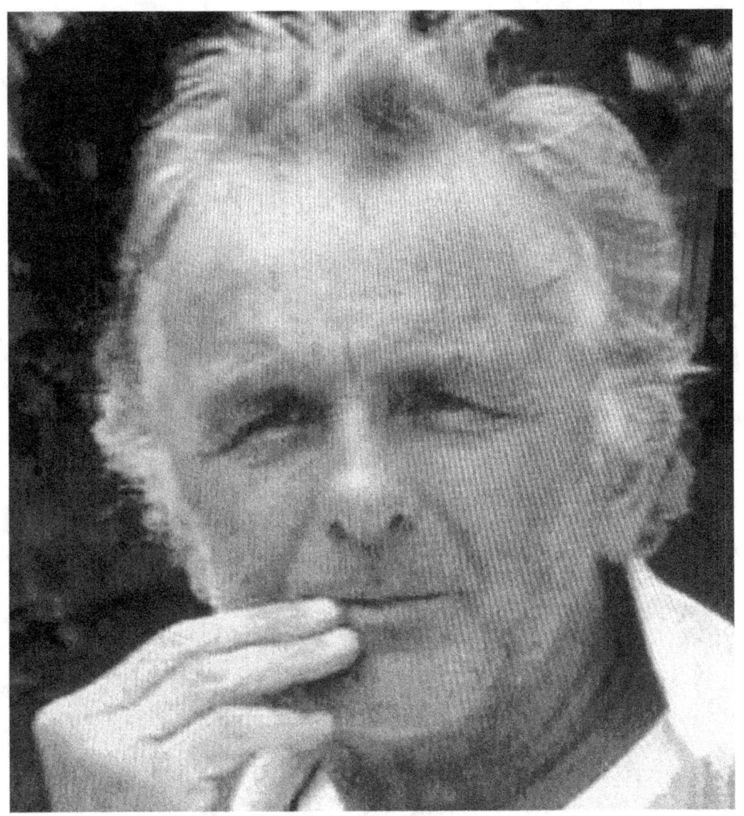

One of my better older photos with hair!

16
THE COOPERS AND HEART DISEASE

'M NOT GOING TOO FAR BACK into the history of the Coopers and am only going to comment on the last few generations. Heart disease within the Cooper men is unbelievably rife and my grandad died of a heart attack in the 60s. For us still-alive men in my family, it doesn't sound good, but it is what it is. From the last generation we lost Big

Frank to a heart attack, then his brothers, Jimmy, Kenny and David have all gone through the trauma of a triple bypass. Sadly, Jimmy is no longer with us, but, with the exception of Big Frank, the Cooper men with dodgy tickers still seem to reach a ripe old age.

So, on that note its fingers crossed for me. Haha, I am laughing to myself.

I recently returned to F6, my old ward in May 2018, where another cousin, Graham Cooper was on stand by for a triple heart bypass. The Cooper Curse strikes again. On my visit I bumped into Daryl, the male nurse. He was still chirpy and smiling. I also bumped into the gentle old guy representing The Ticker Club who was politely going about his business of reassuring patients, whether before or after their operation.

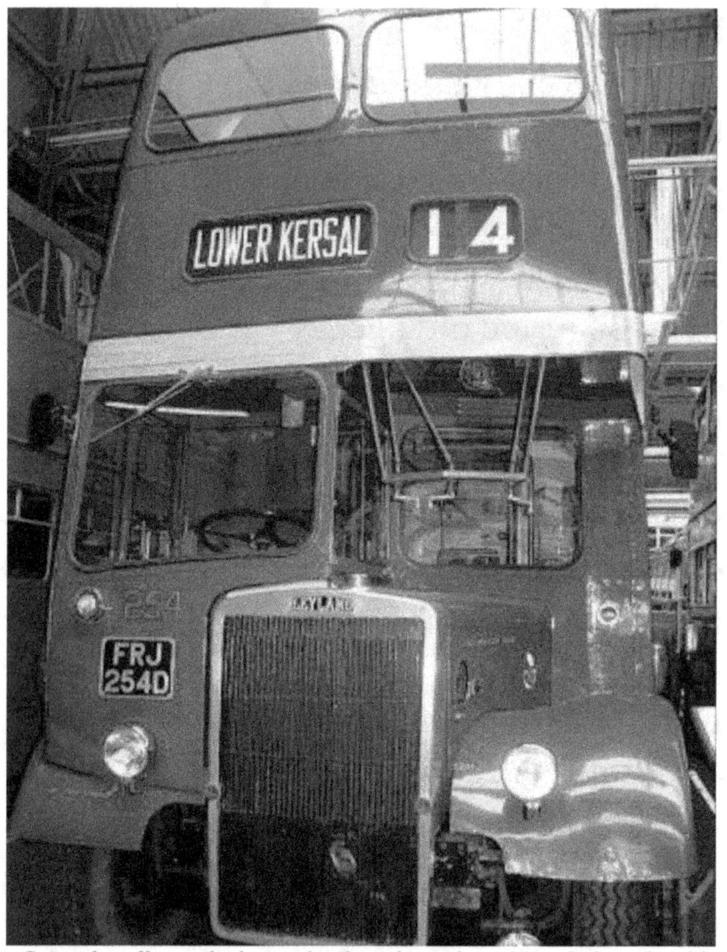

Coincidentally, my lucky number has always been 14 and I love the old double decker buses.

17
THE TICKER CLUB

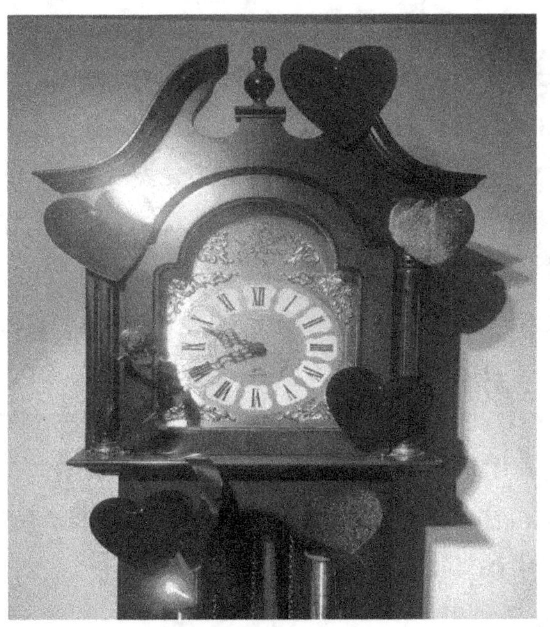

THE TICKER CLUB IS BASED IN Wythenshawe at the Wythenshawe Hospital.

They have their office within the building that is key to the heart wards. It is a charity that's hell bent on supporting people who either are about to have, have had, or are in need of aftercare from heart surgery. It is run by volunteers and relies solely on membership fees, fundraising activities and donations to help in the purchase of much needed equipment and to assist patients. Though I am a member and contribute with a yearly subscription, it is my intention to help raise funds towards their cause and give a little back for the help I received.

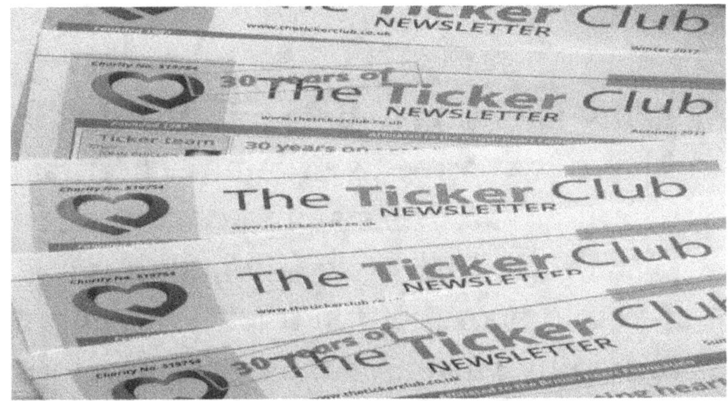

The Ticker Club's quarterly newsletters.

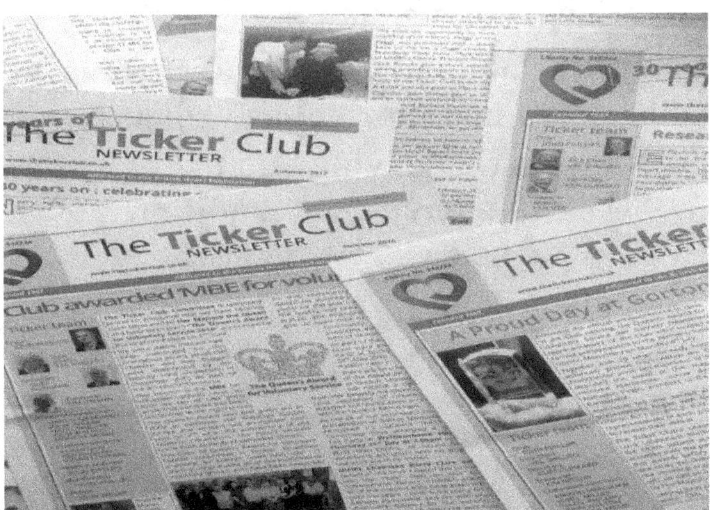

The newsletter keeps all its members up to date on present, past and future activities.

It is my intention to help raise funds and I have two projects in mind. The first is a CD of a Christmas song I wrote called *It's Christmas Time*. The CD includes a lot of versions of the title track, performed by various artists – from solo singers to a choir – and even boasts a Gregorian chant version performed by Father Michael. Other versions include an acoustic and instrumental as well as a karaoke version, leaving you the purchaser to do your own rendition.

The album will be available on Tunecore for downloading from 2023 onwards.

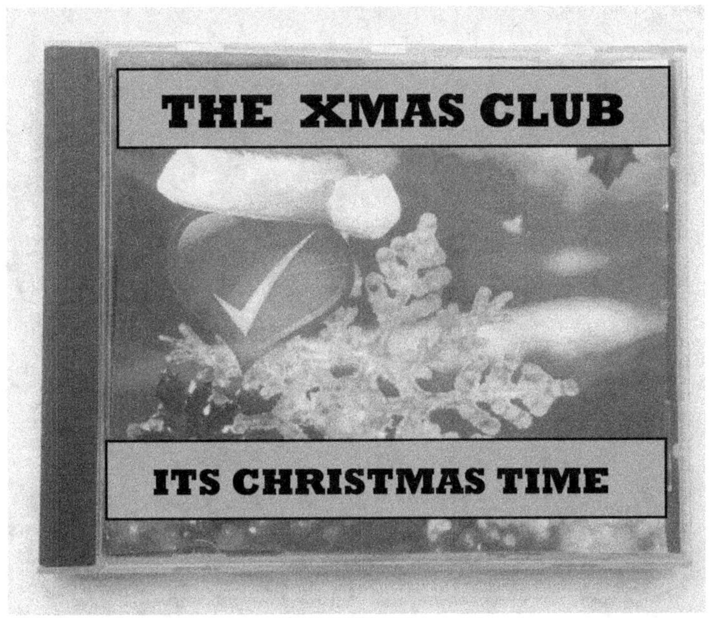

THE CD COVER

'It's Christmas Time'
by The Xmas Club

The Xmas Club is the name given to the collective band of artistes who all gave their time, free of charge, to record the many versions of 'It's Christmas time'.

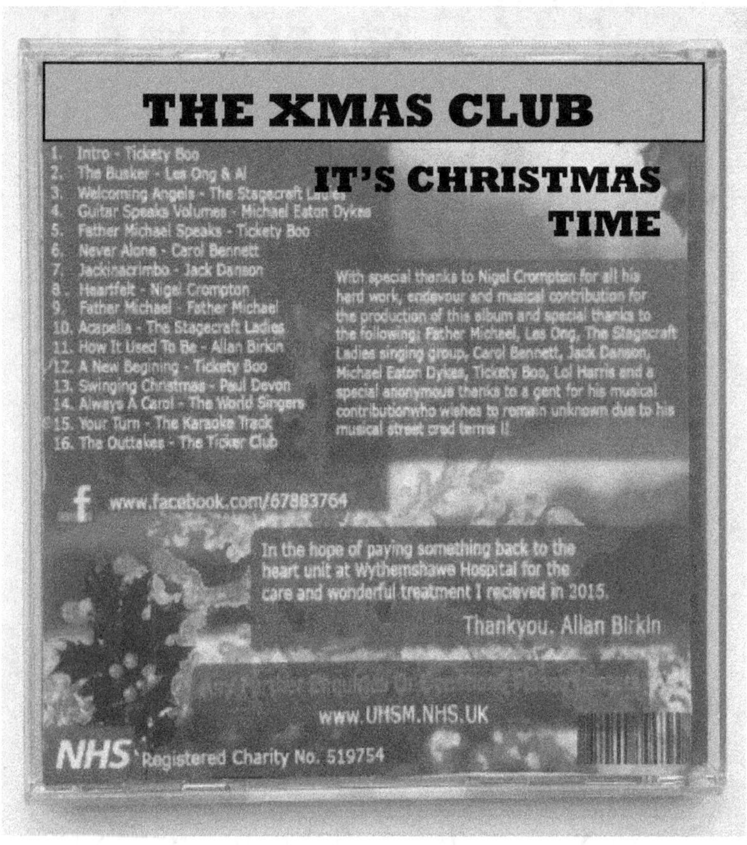

IT'S CHRISTMAS TIME BY THE XMAS CLUB.
THE CD'S REVERSE COVER.

"IT'S CHRISTMAS TIME" BY THE XMAS CLUB

Choirs of angels are singing.
Snow is falling to the ground.
Lights are flashing. Bells are ringing.
Children waiting for the sound
Father Christmas down the chimney.
Leaving presents by the tree
From his sack where there's so many
And the one for you and me is

(Chorus)
Christmas time makes you happy.
Christmas time is full of cheer.
All through life it's been tradition,
And it comes just once a year.
It's Christmas time.

Mince pies, chocolate logs and crackers.
Sleigh bells, reindeers, snowmen too.
When the yuletide season comes around
There is just so much to do.
Take some holly. Take some ivy.
Sneak a kiss under mistletoe.
Eating Christmas pudding, turkey
What's the secret? I don't know at...
(Chorus)

My second project to help raise funds is this book, *Last Day Back in the Room*. It is a blow-by-blow account of my time leading up to the discovery of my heart diagnosis to the operation and what happened afterwards. All the proceeds now and forever will go direct to the funds of The Ticker Club. Fingers crossed it may make the charity a good few pounds. The book, as you may well know if you are reading this, is available on Amazon.

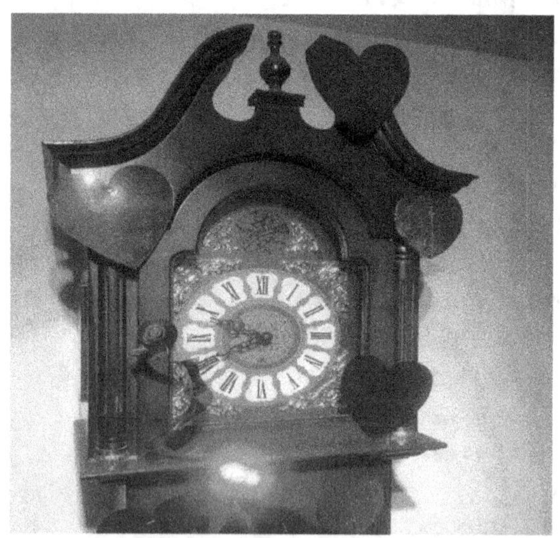

The 'Last Day' clock.

18
OUR STEVE

OUR STEVE, MY BROTHER, was born with a hole in his heart. Although we knew that he had it, and had an operation to correct it, I never knew much about his operation nor did we ever talk about it until I had had my operation. Then, in a phone conversation, I was able to find out most of the details. At this moment in time, we don't see eye to eye. We haven't done for several years nor do I think we probably ever will again. As they say, in life you can choose your friends but you cannot choose your family.

Our Steve was only about seven or eight when he had the operation that left him with a large W-shaped scar on his chest. That would have been likely in the 1970s and technology has moved on so much since then. God knows how difficult an operation or the recovery process was way back then. I know only too well how difficult a job a heart operation is today, and how challenging the recovery process is for a 50-odd-year-old adult. So, I cannot begin to imagine how difficult that was for a seven-year-old child or how the parents with six other children to look after, with jobs to do and a house to run, managed to cope. I suppose it's just like all things in the olden days. You just got on with it and did the best you possibly could.

Because we never spoke about it, we never realised how much he both remembers or coped with it all at such a young age, or even what my nanna and granddad went through. He was their first-born grandchild and boy did they worship the ground that lad walked on. On talking to our Steve, he seemed to remember quite a lot. He remembered dealing with similar things to those I endured - not being able to raise his hands to switch a light on or off was one. He also remembered my mam and dad always being around at the hospital.

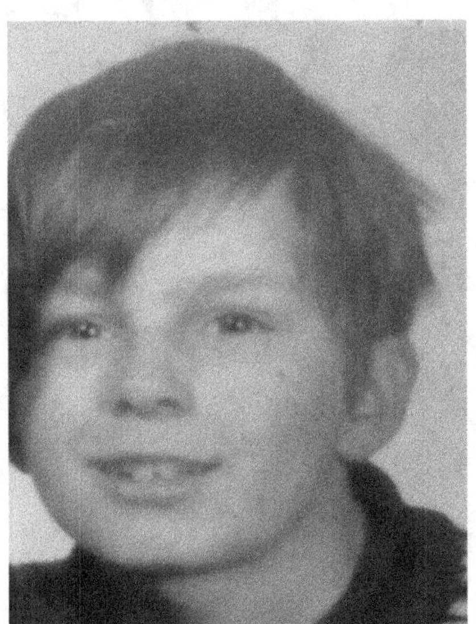

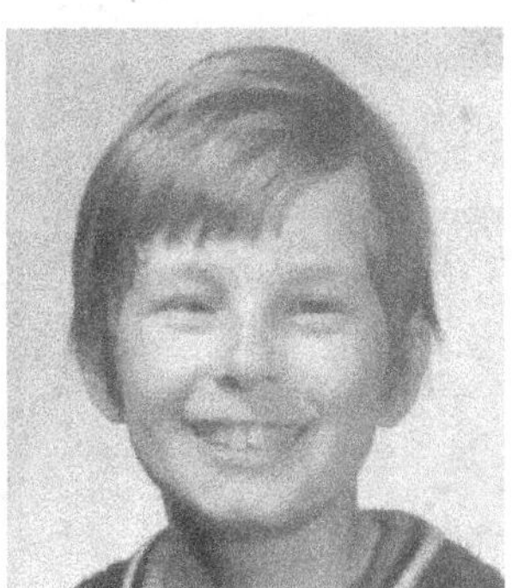

Our Steve after the operation.

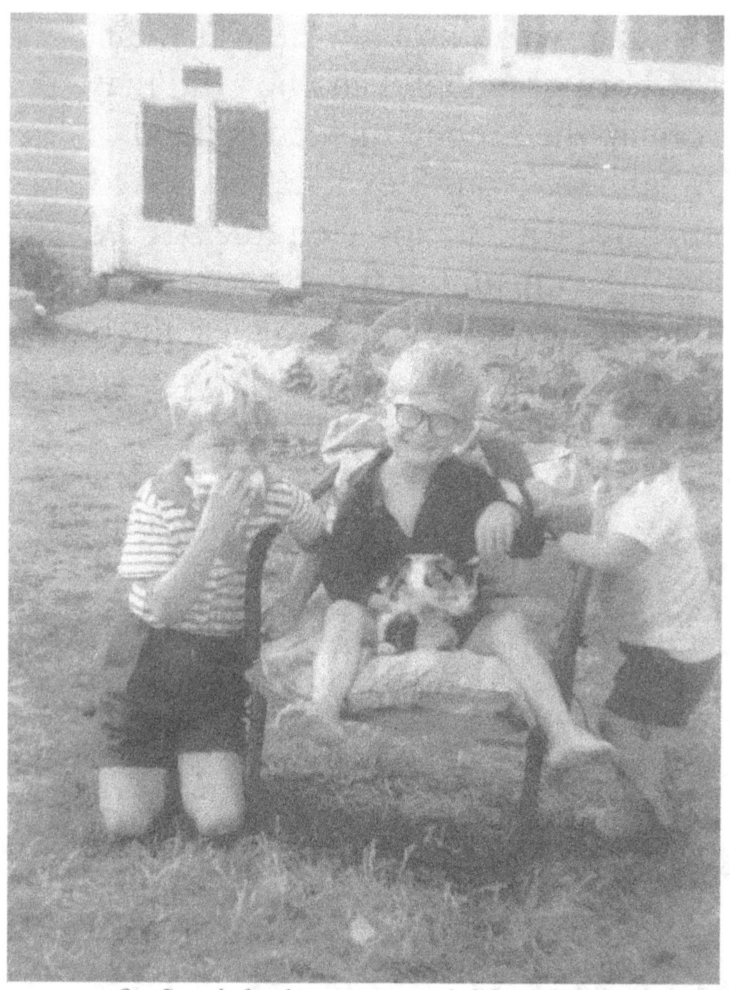

Our Steve before his operation on holiday in Wales.

In just ten minutes of conversation, I was able to discover more than I knew in the whole of the 48 years since his operation. I'm amazed at how much he actually remembered, but then I never forgot the horrors of a trip to the dentist and having gas, so I can understand that bit. Steve recalled needing help to function and needing time to heal. He also spoke of the psychological factors and mental health. Testament to that, in his later life he has suffered from alcohol and substance abuse, and had mental health issues. All, or maybe a few of those issues likely came from the scars of an operation at such a young age. He spoke of the visits to the clinic, his final meeting with the doctor, and the pressure that mum and dad were under. All of us at home were oblivious to that. He also spoke of a respect for life, and recalled that when having the op all the doctors looking in from the outside of theatre. He also recalled having 52 stitches the size of twigs. He said he cringed at the thought of the nurse picking them out one by one. He also spoke of the four-month absence from school and the teachers bringing him work home to do, and also not being able to play out.

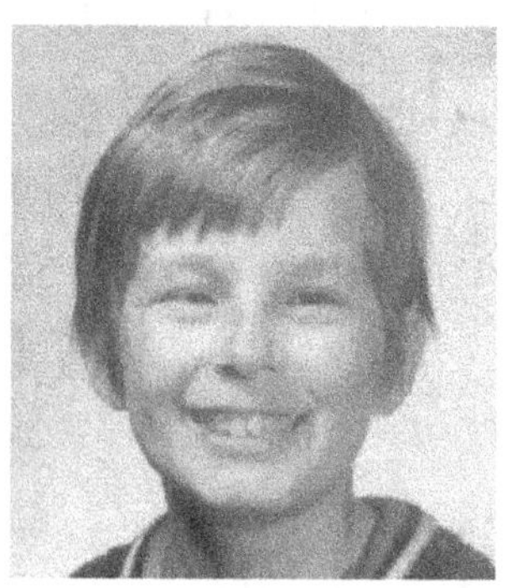

Our Steve.

SAM LEES

I've never spoken to anybody else who has had a mechanical valve fitted, other than the people who were in the hospital at the same time as me, but I was reminded by my son that his old schoolfriend, Sam Lees went through the process almost 14 years ago while he was at school. Almost 11 years ago, he did a few days-work for me and was a proper grafter. I think it was mentioned at the time but, because I had no idea of it all, I suppose I didn't really take much notice. When I think back now, had I have realised how big and serious an operation it was, I may have been a bit less reluctant to put him through the paces. I have been trying to pin Sam down for a little chat but, like all youngsters, it would be easier finding Lord Lucan riding around on the back of Shergar. Or, putting it in footballing terms, getting a lazy player to have a good game or put a shift in. Or, in even more footie-terms as to how I'm feeling at this moment about my favourite team... getting José Mourinho to crack a smile or Romelu Lukaku to score a sitter. Aaaaaarrrrrrgggggghhhhhh, stop it, I'm drifting off the subject now.

<u>19</u>
CHESSY

IN SUMMARY, I DID AND DO feel that my hospital experience was like a brush with death. Here's another that's not dissimilar to my experience. I have a friend who didn't have the same problem as myself, but he did have one of his own. Here is…

…Michael Chester's interpretation of his own experience.

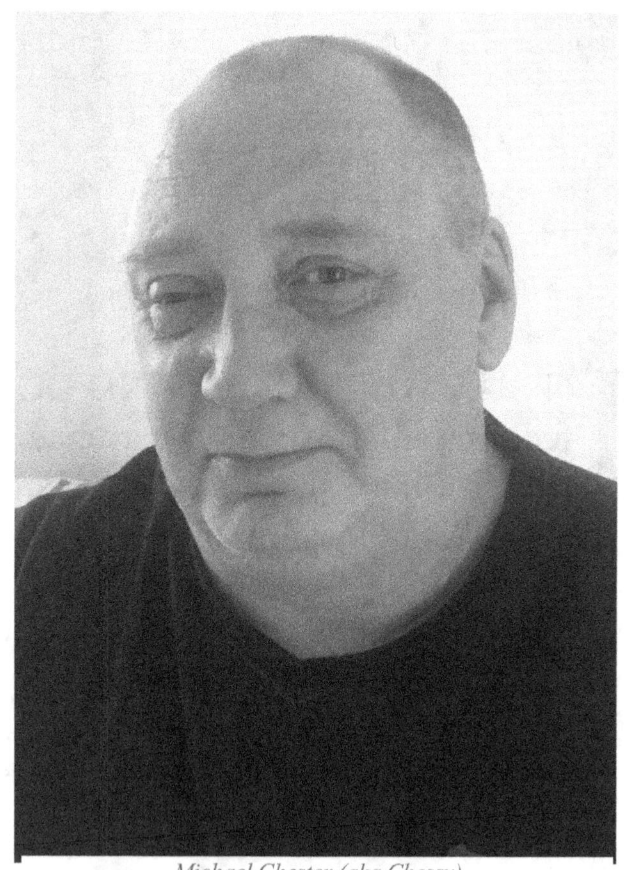

Michael Chester (aka Chessy)

TO THE MOON AND BACK

Hi there my name is Michael Chester (Chessy).

I'm 57 years old and feel very privileged to still be here and able to tell my story.

I will pull no punches. I'm not exactly what you call a centrefold or an Adonis. I carry around with me a few extra pounds, have only one fully-functioning eye and a few of my teeth spend nights in a glass.

To add to that little tale, I've spent a good few years doing both illegal substance and alcohol abuse, I've done very little exercise, had a poor diet and lack of regular sleeping patterns. This, tied in with a big heart and good sense of humour basically sum me up to a 'T'. And, basically, that's me, known to many as... Chessy!

I'm the proud father of three fantastic children: Katie, Liam and Jade (Jade is the youngest at eight years old).

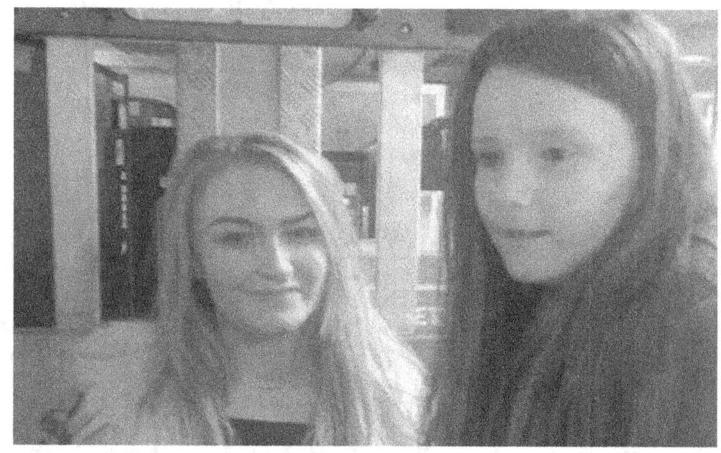

Katie and Jade.

Liam.

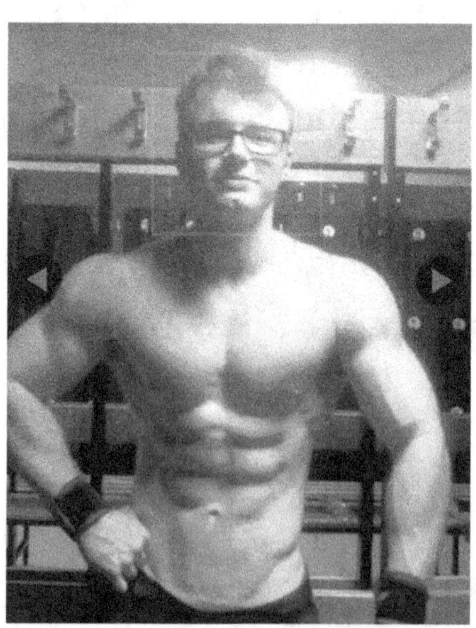

In 2016, I was caught majorly short, and almost wasn't here to tell my tale. In a nutshell, I was given a second chance.

If you've ever remotely gone through a similar experience to me then you too may realise how lucky you are to still be here – as I truly am.

If, like me you are similar in having the same want as I do (to give a little back), then hopefully my little story will spurn you on to complete your task.

So, my story started with an excruciating pain in my shoulder. My 150-year-old doctor decided Zapain was my best plan of attack. He really is a dinosaur and should have retired before I left school.

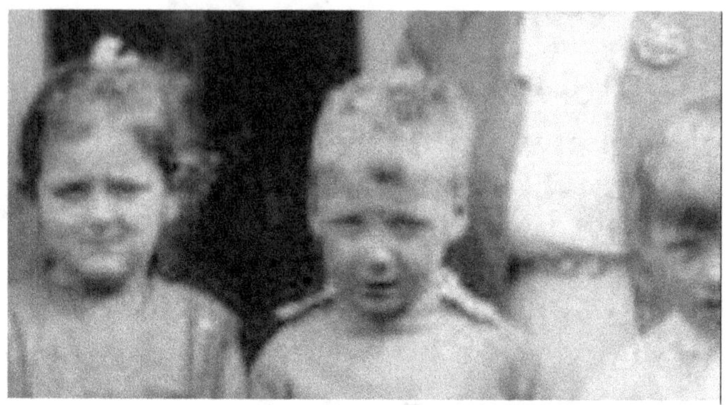

Michael Chester at school.

But beggars can't be choosers. To add to the Zapain, I wasn't in a good place either. I was a little depressed and still downing the good stuff. To top it all off, I ended up constipated. Even listening to my best mate, Anthony Denton's legendary ghost stories couldn't stir my bowels. A full five days later the shoulder pains were now fuelling my stomach pains which in turn led to my blood being poisoned. An ambulance was called and I was rushed to Hope Hospital. The poisoning of my blood led to the thoughts of gallstones, but in truth it did lead me to states of delirium. I was not only a danger to myself but to all those people that were around me attempting to get me better. Because of the delirium I wasn't sure where I was what was happening or basically who I was. I ripped out all the wires and leads that were keeping me functional, which also led to me having to have my meat and two veg stitched back together. For my own and everybody else's safety, they put me in a padded room. My blood poisoning was leading to major organ failure and the hospital were left with no choice but to put me into an induced coma.

I lay in that coma totally unawares for a whole two weeks. I did remember just ever so slightly my eldest daughter being by my side and willing me to get better. I actually felt like I was in a capsule on a journey to the moon and back, and coincidently, when I awoke from my coma and spoke to Katie over the phone,

she asked me the question, "Where have you been?" My answer was simple...
"To the moon and back".

When I looked into the mirror I thought, "Oh my God!" I'd lost almost three stones, my skin was yellow in colour and my eye and teeth were still somewhere languishing in my living room. I immediately phoned Anthony. "Get to my house. Find and bring me my eye and teeth!" It sounds like a sitcom, but I had to make myself look a little more respectable and presentable for any forthcoming visitors. I told Ant I had no idea where anything was so just keep your eye out… haha. I did have a slight giggle to myself as I pictured Ant looking for my eye.

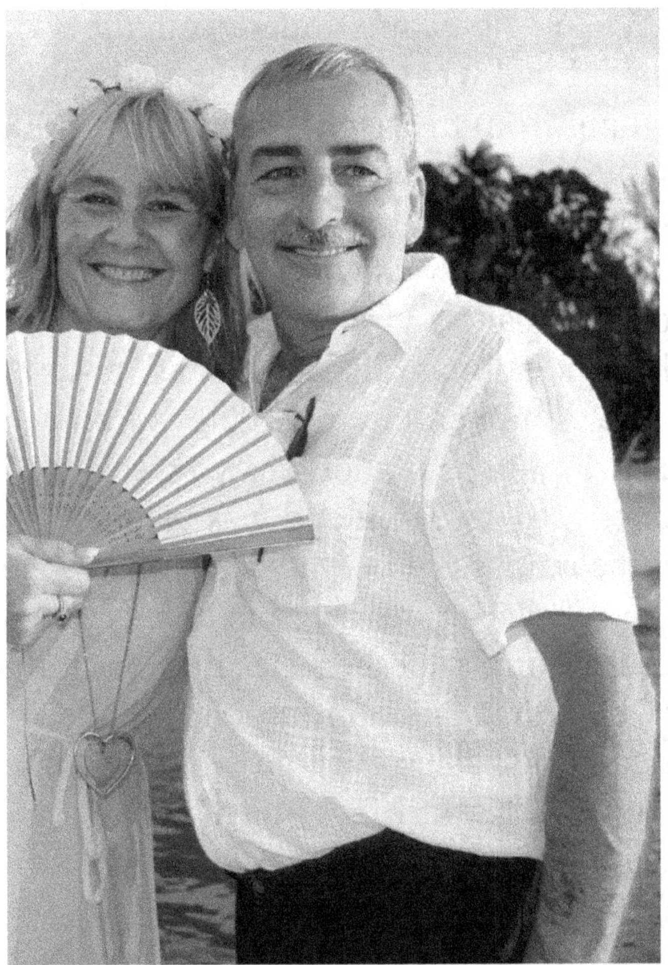

Chessy's long-time good friend, Anthony Denton.

When I first came round from the coma, I had what seemed like two bolts coming from my neck. These were moved to my chest. Apparently, they were doing dialysis on my kidneys that were under-functioning. I was led to believe that the hospital made a virus to fight off the blood poisoning (also known as sepsis) that was preventing my kidneys from repairing. I spent another two weeks on the critical care unit and was taken aback by the amount of people surrounding me who, similar to me, were in comas of one description or another. Because of all that my body had been through, I had to relearn the basics even down to walking again. All in all, I feel I have been very fortunate to have been cared for and looked after by so many people. I couldn't apologise enough to all those who helped me and as a special thank you to the hospital I have volunteered my services, as not only a way of paying something back, but also because it is something I really want to do. My eyes are open wide at the minute. I feel that if an opportunity for part-time employment came up at the hospital, I would grab it with both arms.

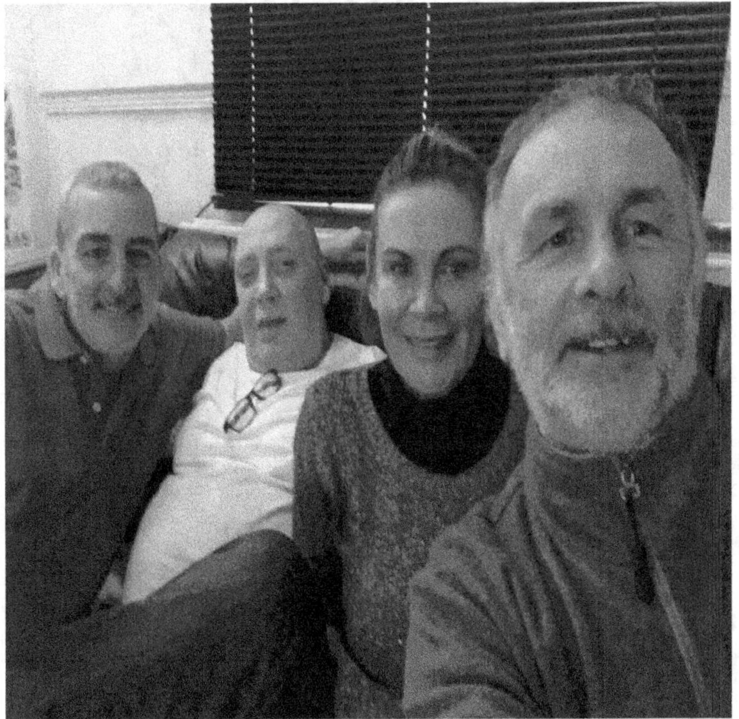

Anthony Denton, Mike Chester, Ann Jones and, Allan Birkin in a good old selfie.

All the best, Chessy.

20
JAMES FRANK
PARKIN

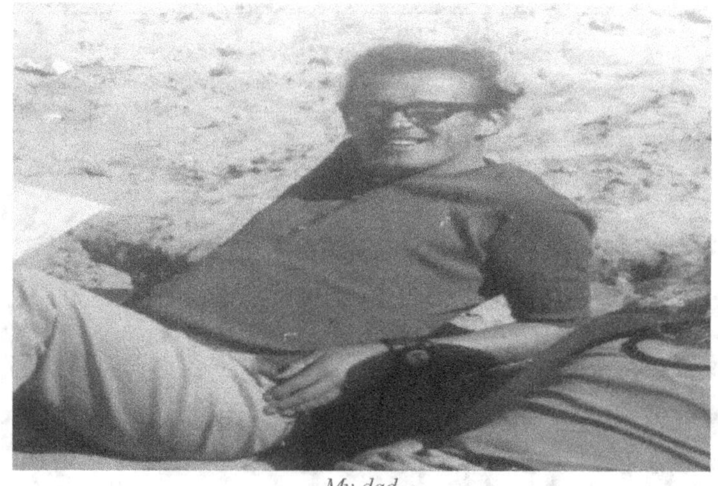

My dad.

James Frank Parkin was born 23/11/1934 and was the first of two sons to James and Amelia Parkin and brother to Kenneth.

He left school and joined the army before meeting my mother in 1961/62 he took on me and my sister and fathered a further five brothers and sisters. We lived on Gallimore Street, Lower Broughton before moving to Lower Kersal in 1970.

My dad was a bricklayer by trade and worked for Harry Lomas Builders on Tenerife Street, Lower Broughton.

He did many of what we term as foreigners (jobs for cash) and, as I got older, he used to take me with him for my first taste of the building industry.

He was a special man who was kind, loving and asked for very little in return. He enjoyed combing his thinning hair before departing for the last half hour at The Castle pub, he worked many a job for the Jewish community and never failed to bring home a bag of Jewish treat cakes and biscuits. Lovely jubbly. He drove the most modest of cars, but in all the years he spent driving he never held a full license! When I found out, it made sense why every time he passed a copper the colour used to drain from his face. The police weren't as on the ball as they are in this day and age, and besides that it's all on computer now so you can't get away with anything...

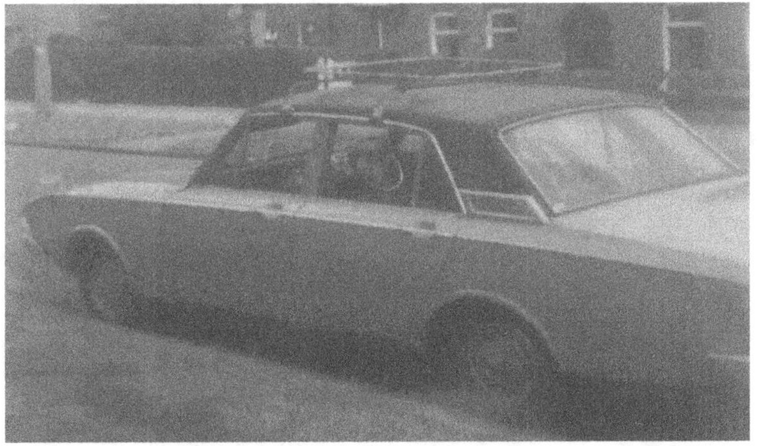

Dad's green Corsair!

One funny story... He sold his green corsair to a chap called Thompson who on the same day as the purchase, crashed it whilst drunk right outside our very house, then dumped it and did a runner. What are the chances? Everybody thought my dad had crashed the car.

He eventually got a maintenance job at CPC in Trafford Park, helped by his good friend, Albert Jamieson. It was a good number - not too hard and with better rewards. We may not have been a wealthy family but we always had a holiday and good Christmases. Although I loved going to Wales, my best ever holiday was our week-long trip to Butlins in Skegness. Nanna and grandad came too. Everything there was free.

The song that reminds me most of that trip was *The Hustle* by Van McCoy. To this day I get Goosebumps on hearing that intro. There was a lot of activity at Butlins and I made the most of all on offer, including the girls. I entered a fancy dress talent competition and here's me doing my Charlie Chaplin impression in my grandad's clothes.

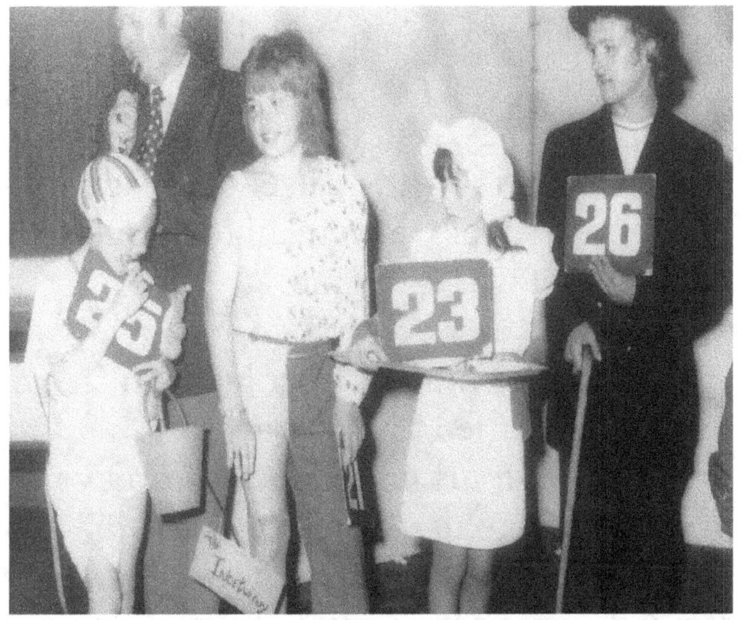

Number 26, me in my Charlie Chaplin clothes.

I left home in 1978/79. At that point, my family still lived in Kersal, but soon afterwards left for Swinton in 1981/82.

Dad's illness started soon after that. His wife (my mother) left him for another man, and that was it. He was ill and a broken man to boot. We were forever toing and froing to the doctors but not once did they say to us at any point that he wasn't getting better but was on a downhill slope of no return. Had his seven still-young children known that fact perhaps we may well have made his last couple of years a little easier and happier. It's so sad. I feel we were all too young to realise what was going on.

He passed away on May 24th 1984, two years and four months after his own father. We buried him at Agecroft Cemetery, but his mother never forgave us nor spoke to us again. She wanted her son cremating. If I'm honest, I don't remember the argument, but then I don't remember a lot.

I wrote a song titled *J.F.P.* as a special tribute to my dad, James Frank Parkin, a true gent, great father and a very nice man just like his own father, my grandad, who went by the same name, James Parkin.

J.F.P.

There's only one world and into it you came
To raise a family was your greatest aim
You worked eight days a week all the hours god send
When we were out of order you put us right on the mend

J.F.P. we owe you the world
Cos you looked after us all and you never got returned
The whole of our family we all feel sad
Were all growing up and miss the good times we had
You were treated so wrong in a way I hope where you've gone
Something good comes along because you deserve the best J.F.P.

Until it's too late we don't appreciate
Life flies by at such an incredible rate
Now you're not here and we just couldn't say
How much you were right in your own little way.

In a way you're lucky its worse left behind
The pain is so hard and the torments a grind
We know where you've gone and we'll never forget
We'll catch up with you one day just to pay off our debt.

J.F.P., we owe you the world
Cos you looked after us all and you never got returned
The whole of our family we all feel sad
Were all growing up and miss the good times we had
You were treated so wrong in a way I hope where you've gone
Something good comes along because you deserve the best J.F.P.

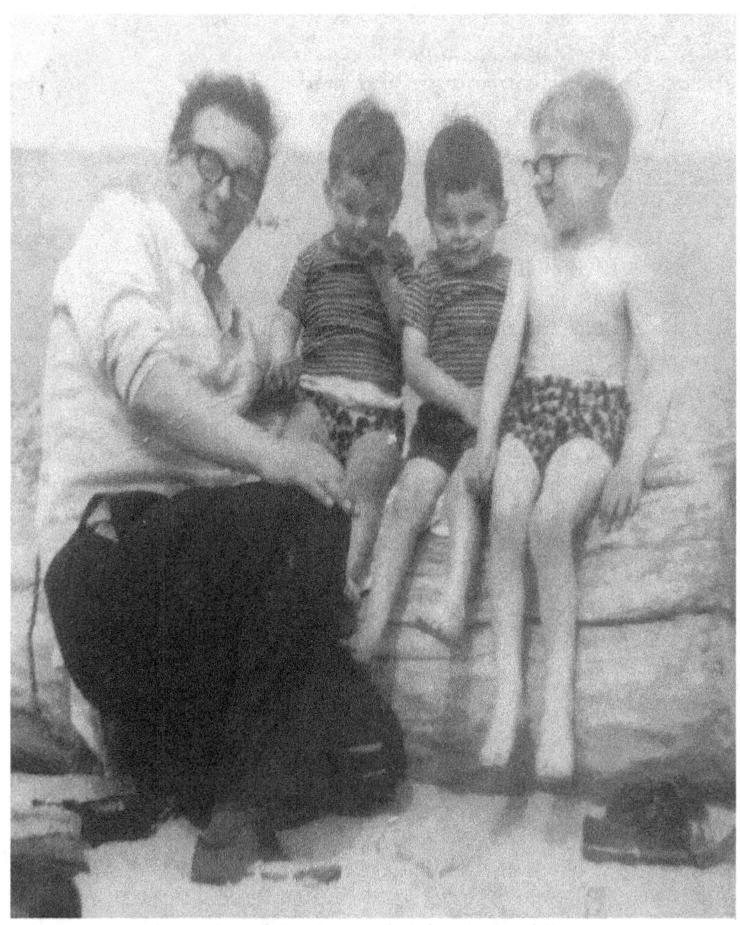

James Frank Parkin, with John, Ian and Steve.

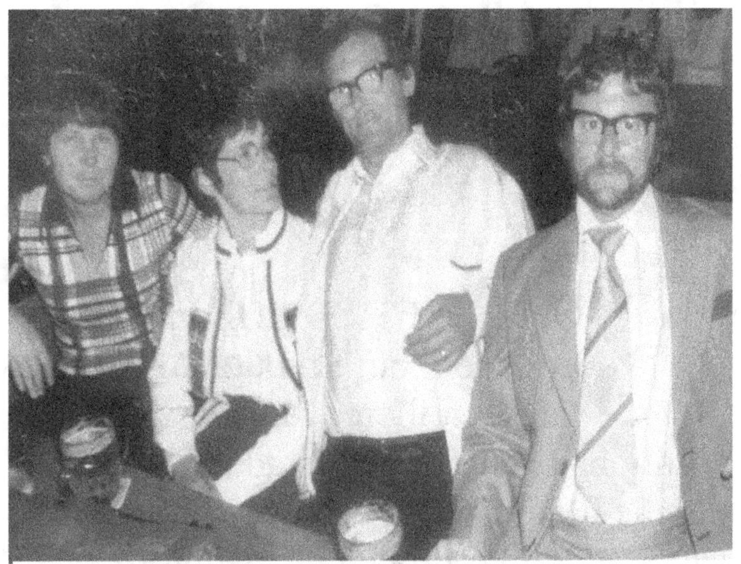

Margaret Daley, Ma, amd Dad and Kenny Cooper.

<u>21</u>
IN ADDITION

S O, I REACHED THE END OF my book, but I thought, in all fairness, there were a few additions I felt obliged to add. Three people I knew who had gone through the same or similar procedure as myself (more or less). So, I decided to include, in their own words, their own versions.

Ladies and Jellybeans, I give you Ged McHugh, Mike Gaynor and last (but no means least), Mr Lawrence Harrison.

GERARD MCHUGH

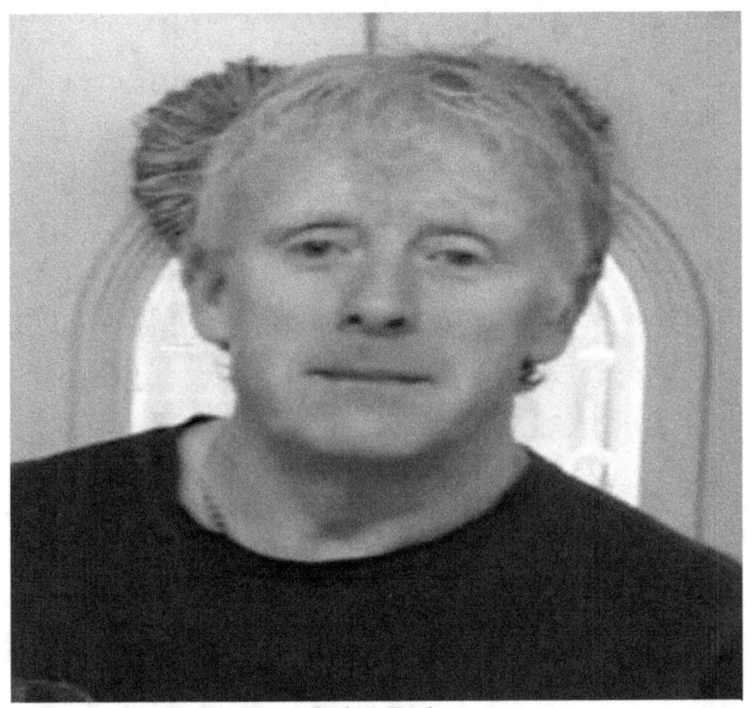

Ged McHugh.

Hello. I was born in November 1969, the eighth of nine children to my mother, Kathleen McHugh (maiden name McLoughlin). When I was two years old, my mother noticed I was not very good with my breathing so she took me to the local doctors. This was Dr Gill on Walkden Road, Walkden, which eventually moved to a new building called the Gill Medical Centre which was apparently named after Dr Gill.

The doctors at the time said I had a bad cold, but my mother was not so sure and she had plenty of first-hand experience, having already raised so many children. I was sent to the hospital for tests where they noticed I had a defective aortic valve. My heart also had several holes. I was educated a little later on in life that most children are born with holes in their hearts. Apparently by the ages of seven or eight, more have repaired themselves, but, because of my faulty valve, my holes failed to repair themselves. This was what caused me to be breathless especially when I walked up and down the stairs. This made me go pale in the face and weak.

While I was on the NHS monitor list, I received many check-ups at Gartside Street in Manchester. I also went to Pendlebury Children's Hospital once a year for examinations from trainee doctors. They would tell the main doctor what their thoughts were regarding my heart. I didn't mind this because, for my time and trouble, they used to give me £5. Being a young lad, £5 was a lot of money!

I left school with an O level in joinery, and this was what I needed to go on a CITB training course. I was placed at Salford University. In those days, you would do six months in college then six months on site. I learnt all the joinery skills; skirtings, architraves, doors, windows, roofs and all the other jobs that enabled me to become a qualified joiner. I was advised against this type of work as a long-term career because of the strenuous work involved. So, I opted for a much lighter and easier role as a CAD technician. Again, I had to attend college to train but, to this day, that remains my employment as I work alongside the Highways England in maintaining the motorway network across the country.

Going back a little, it wasn't till I reached the ages of 16/17 that I went back to Gartside Street where they decide I had grown enough to warrant the major operation needed on my valve. My operation was in October 1997, but prior to that I had to attend several times for procedures which included (under local anaesthetic) having a camera inserted into my arm. I was able to watch on a screen and get a close-up view on the condition and working procedure of my aortic valve.

The operation itself was performed at Wythenshawe Hospital. It took six hours, after which I was placed in the ICU unit for a couple of days.

I had pain and was very sore. One of the main reasons was that to get to the heart they have to cut the sternum bone.

They also don't tell you that you're left with a ticking sound, so I was thinking the doctor had left his watch inside me. It's the sound of the valve working and I'm afraid that noise will stay with me till the end. As the doctors laughingly put it, the time to worry is when you can no longer hear it. In work, I often have acquaintances comment on the ticking but I'm used to it now.

My time spent in hospital was almost two weeks and on my return home I was told to take things easy. I did begin to notice the difference in both my breathing and energy levels. This was proof the aortic valve was the reason behind my earlier difficulties.

When I originally had the operation, I was placed on a drug called sinthrone which has since been replaced with warfarin, and I need to have checks every six to eight weeks. It is a precaution to ensure the blood doesn't get too thick or too thin.

There have been many funny incidents since receiving my valve, but I'm told that as long as I don't overdo it, I should live a long and happy life. One of the funny incidents happened when taking my driving test. The female tester was almost driven round the bend by a constant ticking that she thought was a fault with the car's running functions. I had to tell her it was my heart. Bless her, she passed me, haha.

On one occasion while sat in church, a little boy looked at me and then said to his mother "That man is ticking!" She looked embarrassed and apologised to me. I didn't have the heart to tell her that her son was right.

Since the operation, I've been able to build up my stamina and exercise my

work ethic by swimming and running. I've done several half marathons and also done the Manchester to Blackpool Cycle Run, raising a good few pounds for charity in the process. I'm also proud of the fact I took part in a mini triathalon at Heaton Park. All in all, I am eternally grateful to both my parents, the doctors and the NHS for giving me the opportunity to live as normal a life as the next man.
Thank you,
Ged McHugh.

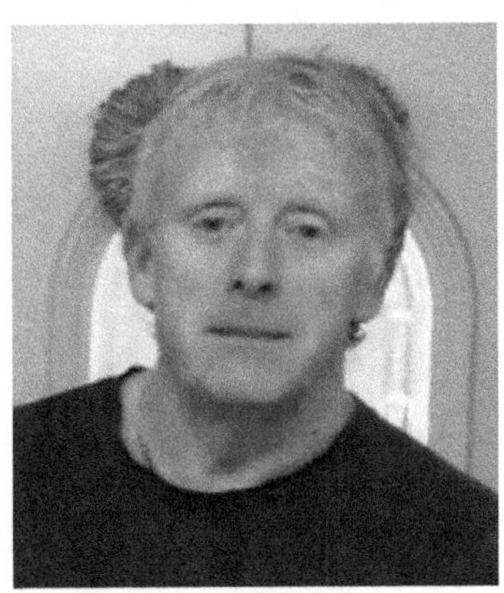

Ged

MIKE GAYNOR

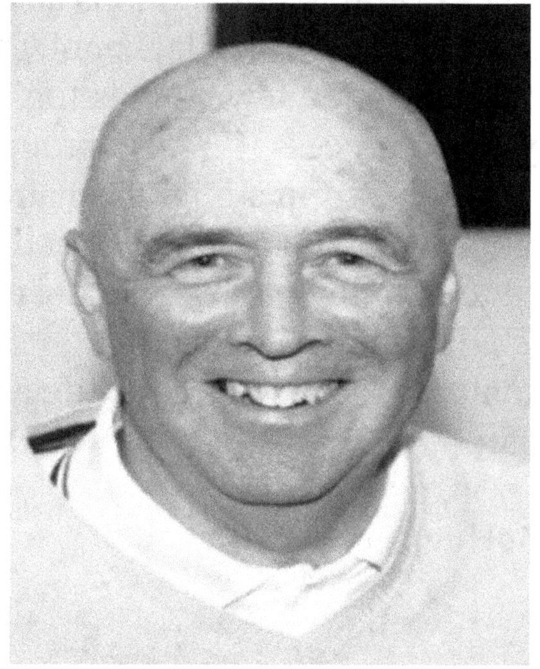

Mike Gaynor.

I suppose the best place to start would be to say that I've never had any health issues, never mind heart issues, and that's in 62 years.

I both played and coached football till I was 50. Then, while rushing and not taking care as I was doing a flagging job, I broke a vertebra. This caused my semi-retirement plus the start of the grief and mither in my home life. I was wanting to graft but found myself unable to.

One year later, I found myself lodging at my sister's. 2018 was turning into a disastrous year. Five months later after my relationship failed, I got a settlement on my house, which enabled me to move on with my life. I bought and moved into a new apartment in 2019 and I was thinking it was the start of a new chapter as everything was going hunky dory. I did still have a little battle with the DWP over a spinal injury that eventually (after several appeals on their decisions) I won my case.

So, time moved on. I went for a nice simple November walk which in turn turned into the start of my nightmare. I'd only walked half a mile but found myself gasping for air with excruciating pains going through my chest, arms and hand. I tried telling myself I would be fine and took a few moments to recover while leaning against the railings.

It wasn't until the following March that I finally got an appointment where they informed me of something important. Between November and March, I had suffered a heart attack. Nine hours later, I was back home with all sorts of thoughts running through my head about what may have caused it. I put it down to life's silent killer – STRESS.

So, my journey began. I was off to Wigan Cardiology for an angiogram and stents. I was thinking it was happy days and that I would be as good as new the following day. I jumped the gun.

My arteries were blocked with calcium. My worst fears were confirmed. My procedure was to be a major heart operation – I was booked in for a bypass.

In January 2022, I got a call from my consultant asking me how I felt after my operation, I told him I hadn't had it yet. To say he wasn't best pleased was an understatement. He was not a happy man. The very next day I got a call with a date for my operation. I was booked in for March 23rd. Prior to all that, I'd been a good lad, avoiding all chances of catching COVID, then, sure as eggs are eggs, I caught it from my pre-op nurse. You couldn't make it up! My operation was put on hold after that first cancellation, for reasons not always mine. I had a further three cancelled dates, and the fourth cancellation was due to the surgeon going on his summer holidays.

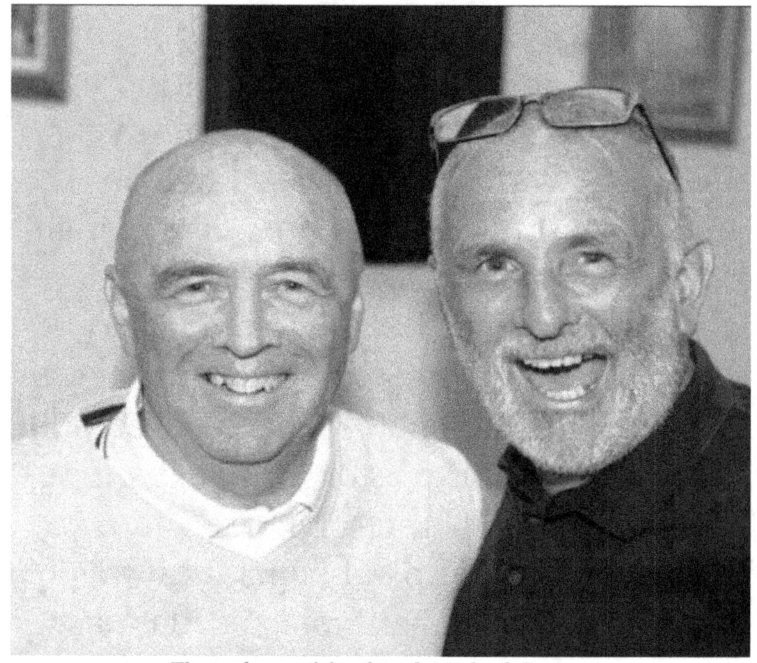

The author and his friend, Michael Gaynor.

I'm not a bad-tempered man, but I decided to show my anger a little and made a complaint. What do you know, within three days I was in and under the surgeon's knife. I had a quadruple bypass in a private hospital and I certainly got the royal treatment. I even got a private plane to and from the hospital. Not really, I'm kidding – still got my sense of humour!

I don't consider myself a lucky man but sensibly, after my angiogram, I wasted no time in changing the diet that may well have accelerated my condition. Red meat was history and I did love a T bone, but after the operation it was fish, chicken and plenty of vegetables. A pint of beer became a distant memory I tried my best to build up my fitness which helped in my doctor signing me off after 13 weeks.

I still have a few aches and pains but, in general, I'm feeling good.

I have two favourite sayings in life. One is "When my eyes don't open in the morning. It is then that I will start to worry" and the second and most important is "I don't have problems, I have solutions" and my tip for anyone who has problems in their life is TALK and don't ever bottle it up...

All the best,
Michael

LAWRENCE HARRISON (LOZZY)

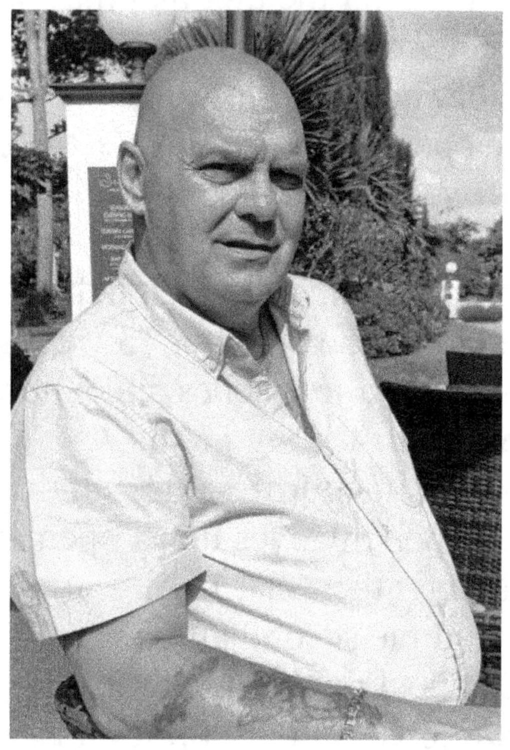

This man is Salford through and through. Salford born and bred. Lawrence Harrison began life in a humble terraced house on Seddon Street off Fredrick

Road, but now is in a place he has lived for almost 60 years. The place he calls home is Lower Kersal.

Lawrence came from a very large family of three sisters and five brothers, so their household was 11 people all contained in a high-rise apartment block (Browning House on Kersal Flats). He came from a very large family and produced a large one of his own with Kim, his wife of almost 44 years. This brought them to well over double figures in the grandparent stakes!

Life hasn't always been easy, yet Lawrence (known as Lozzy to many) seems to have taken it all in his stride. Being the local tough nut as a kid, he spent times in the local boys' homes or as the do-gooders would be quick to point out, Borstal. Loz frequented Manor Heath after the local schools decided he was a little more than a handful and they didn't have the time or patience to put him back on the straight and narrow. When school finished for good it was out into the big bad world to earn a living.

His first job brought him to Platt's Clothiers on Greengate, a works that had an abundance of local people plying their trades to pay their ways in life. It was there that he met his future wife, Kim, a lady who, to this very day, is still by his side and, as tiny as she is, will take no shit from Manor Heath's old tough nut.

Lawrence has gone through life doing various jobs, including a stint at Pilkington's Tiles. He even had a spell as a newsagent. I can certainly vouch for that. He, like myself, also hit the stage as a compere for a stint at the Borough Social Club on Station Road in Swinton.

His employment at present is at the Salford Royal Hospital where he has treaded the boards for many a year. As well as his love for producing offspring, he also had a passion for alcohol, cigarettes and the good old English breakfast. These are what brought him to where he is now – a recovering heart attack victim who endured a quadruple bypass. But, if asked if he has any regrets, the answer would be a firm "No! I wouldn't change a thing. I've lived my life, I've partied well and I'm still going strong at present".

Lozz's health is ticking along nicely but that's not to say the last 4-5 years have been anything but easy.

While going for a morning stroll five years ago, he found himself gasping for breath. This had the doctor sending him to Wigan Infirmary for stents to be fitted.

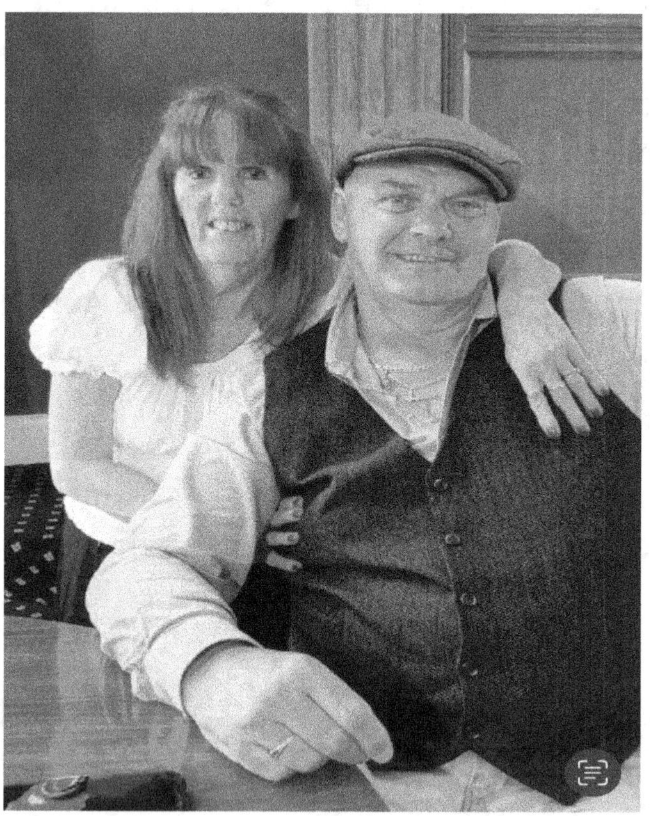

Lozzy and his Mrs… Kim.

While lying there on the hospital bed, the doors burst open and he was summoned to get in the ambulance. He was whizzed over to Wythenshawe Hospital. They suspected then confirmed a heart attack and revealed that emergency treatment was needed. A quadruple heart bypass was on Lozz's agenda.

He will be the first to tell you and admit he was scared of no man, but that statement had him crying like a baby. It was a complete wake-up call. Lozz felt his life couldn't end then and that he had so much to do. He had kids and grandkids that needed their grandad. He was ordered to ditch the cigarettes, lower the alcohol consumption and start taking better care of himself, especially if he wanted to see his beloved Manchester United lift that Premier League trophy ever again!

Apart from a few hiccups along the way, Lawrence is doing fine at present, but when asked the question "Have you anything to say to people?" he came up with the following statement. "Don't ever think you're invincible. If you do you may well be in for a shock." On that statement he takes a puff on his vape cigarette and reminds me he will be meeting up with his brother and drinking partner, Anthony Harrison a little later in the day. But he swears it is only for a couple.

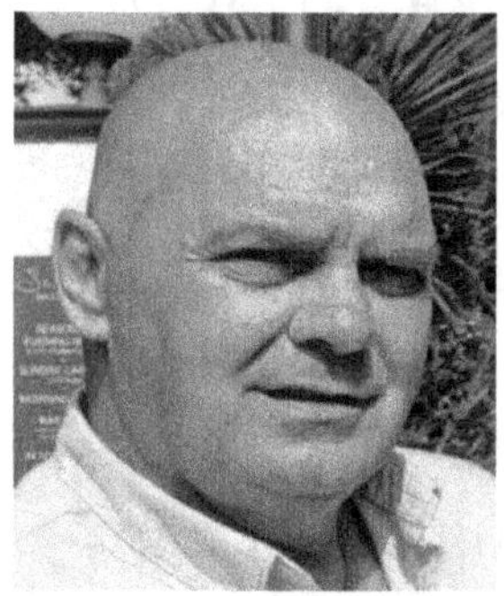

All the best,
Lozzy.

<u>22</u>
ON REFLECTION

So, today is the second week of January 2023 and this is my chance to reflect on everything before this book is put to print. I'm in my ninth year since my operation, and yes, I'm still here, still on medication, still having my A and R levels checked every few months. They check that my ticker is still ticking every 12/18 months. The funny thing is that when I had this valve fitted, they omitted telling me that I'd become a human clock. In the dead of night, I hear every tick. I can sometimes still hear it when surrounded by noise. I have on more than one occasion been asked by someone in the room who doesn't know I've been operated on, "Can you hear that?" "Hear what," I ask. "That ticking?" "Yes." "That will be me." "What? What? Fuck off!"

When I bring their head closer to my chest they are amazed. The truth is though that nobody is more amazed than me. This tick tocks more than 70/80 times a minute, 4800 times an hour. Almost 116,000 times a day. Almost 800,000 a week. In fact, it's a whopping 40 million times a year. Yes, I hear what you're thinking. Me too. I often wonder how I am not in a straightjacket haha. However, I do think of the amazing fact that (so far) something made on planet Earth has (so far) worked a massive third of a billion times.

When I originally planned to write this book, I offered it along with the CD *Its Christmas Time* in order to raise a few funds for The Ticker Club in gratitude for the help they had given me, but after several meetings we became embroiled in red tape and controversial points so I backed away. I decided to do them anyway and just send them any monies made.

Since I started putting the book together, I have come up with a few covers. In fact, there are three in total, before finally finding myself where we are at right now.

I've included all three in the book.

Reiterating a few things I said earlier, we all have a number problem. We have no idea what it is until (without stating the obvious) it is too late. Because, when your number's up it is up for whatever reason. Life is not a rehearsal. You need to do what makes you happy and what keeps you smiling. With a little luck, by the time your number is called you will have left your mark and done exactly what you set out to do.

As is said and quoted by many: "We are only passing through."

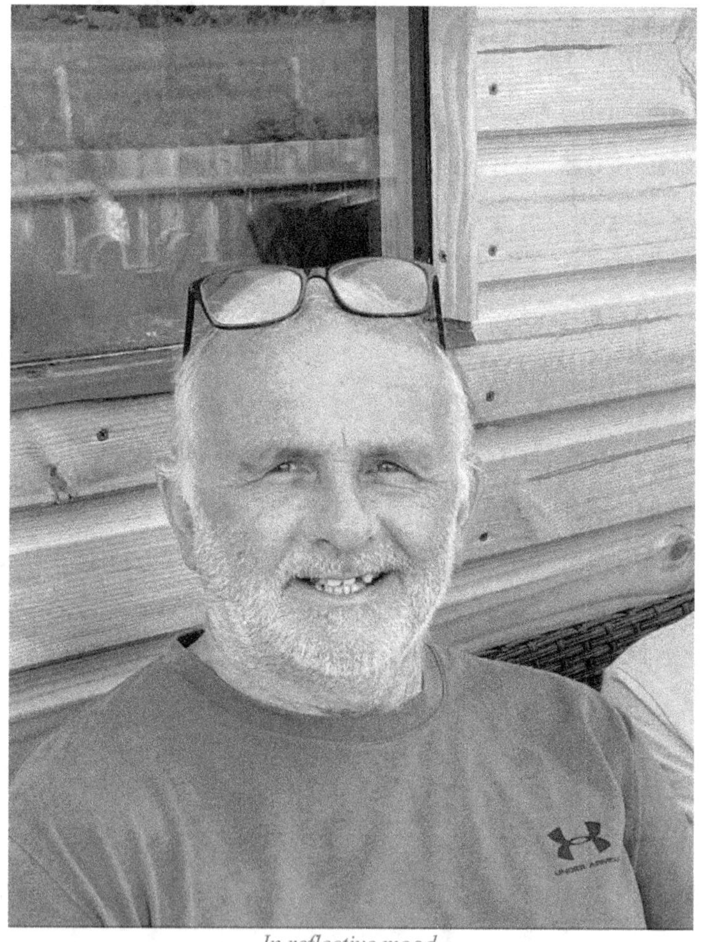

In reflective mood.

It took several ideas for the front cover before we finally settled for the one that adorns this book.

This was the first.

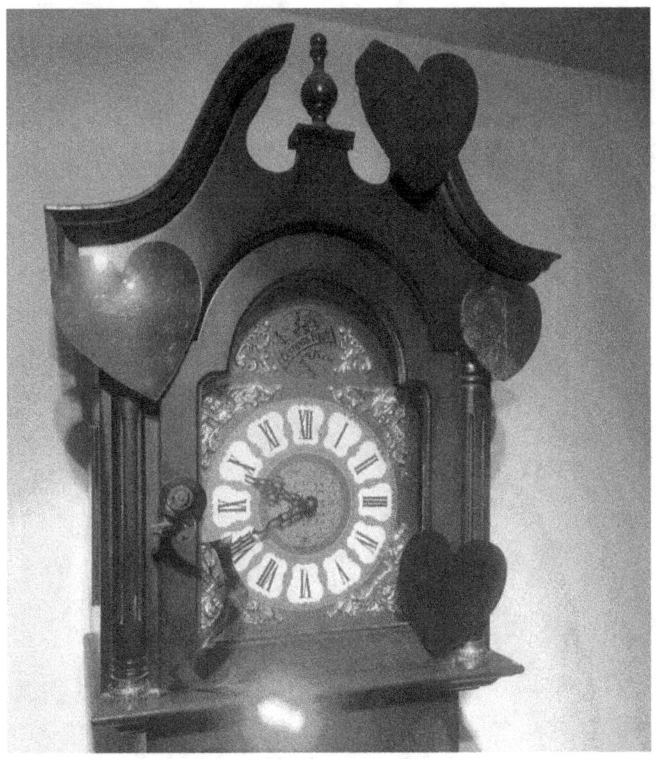

The first cover.

The second.

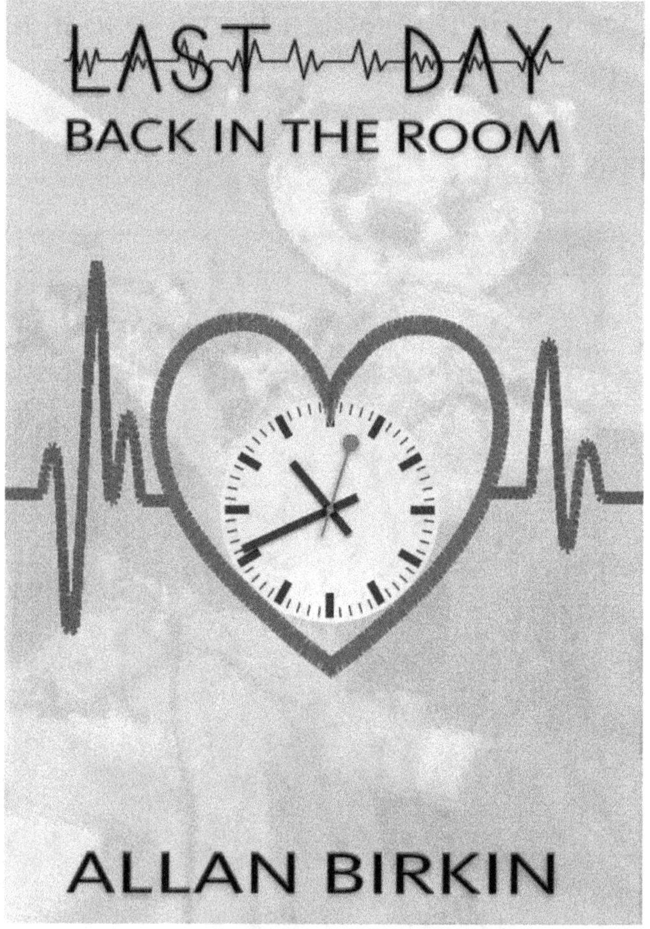

The second considered cover design.

The third.

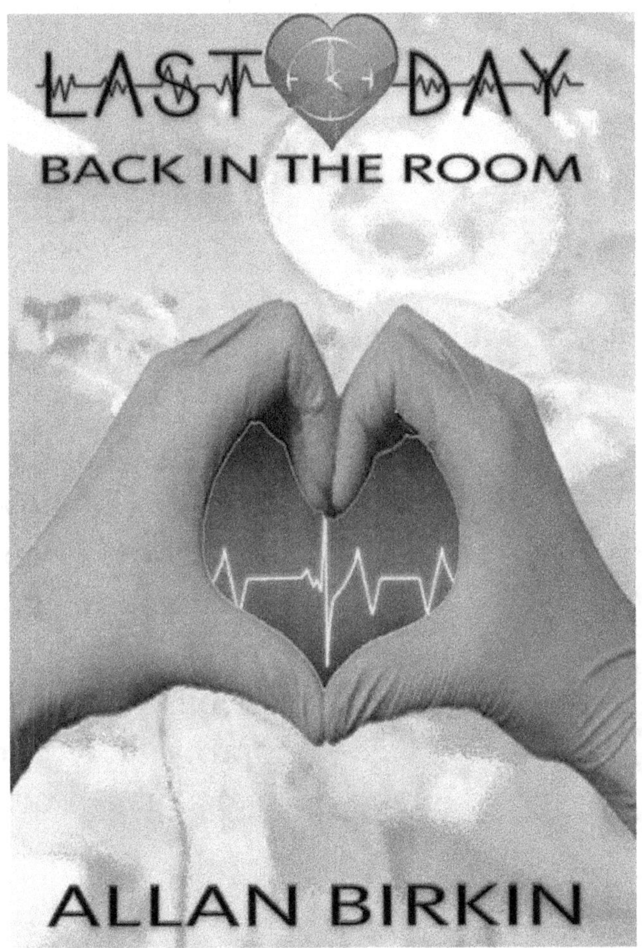

The third considered cover design.

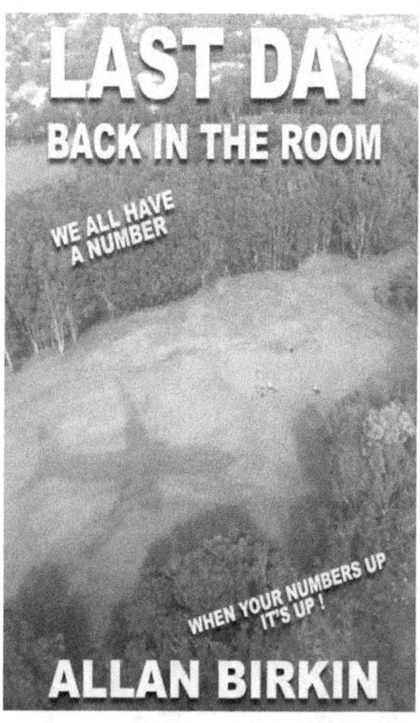

Eventually, I settled for the cover you see here. It is a picture taken by my daughter as she came into land in Australia. It shows the shadow of her plane across a golf course and the green is appropriately shaped as a heart.

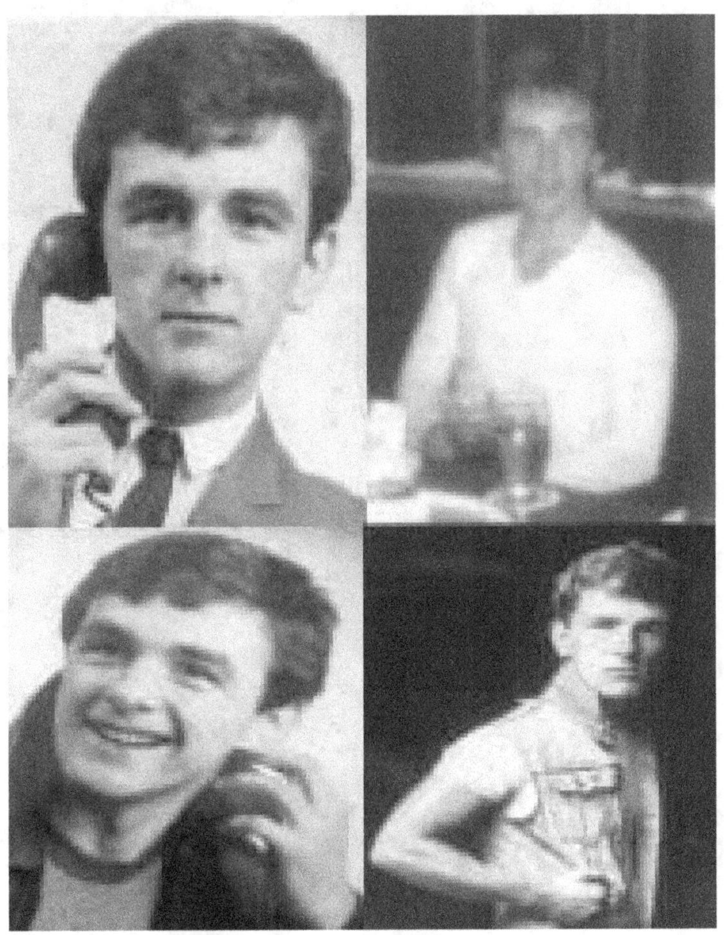

Just a few of my many memories.

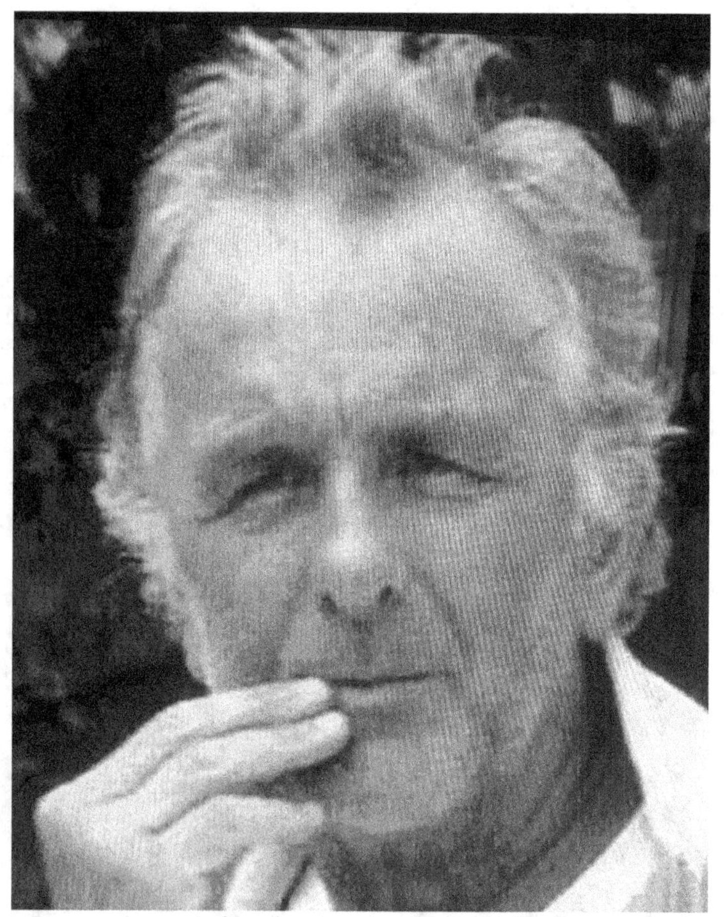

And one last one. Age gets to us all!

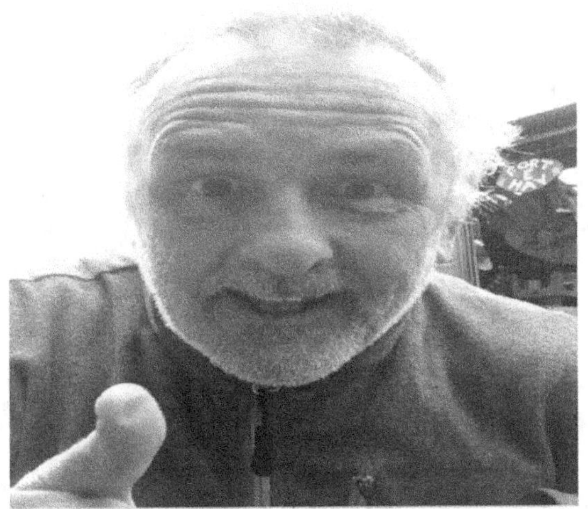

Allan.

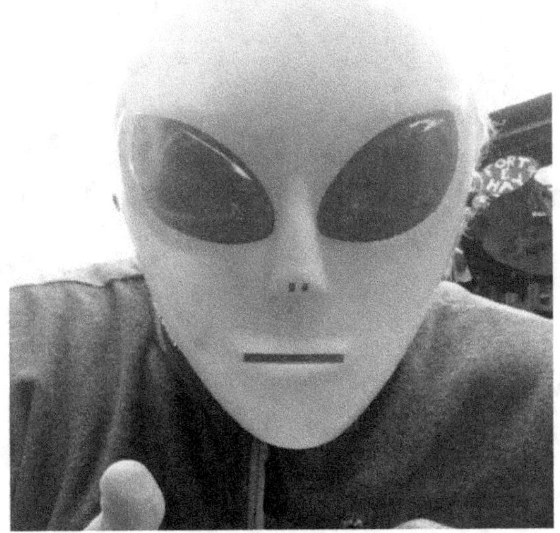

Also, Allan?

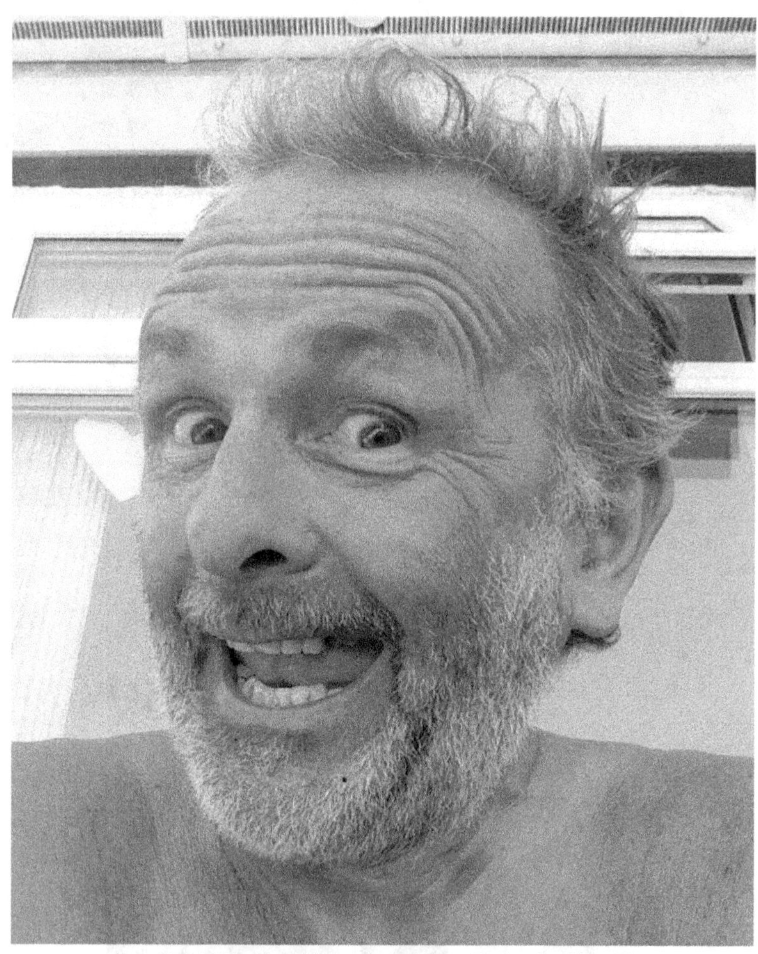

*Allan David Birkin, AKA Adge, Alber, Birky, Scully, Albert,
Spottymolldoon, oh, and Rupert, apparently.*

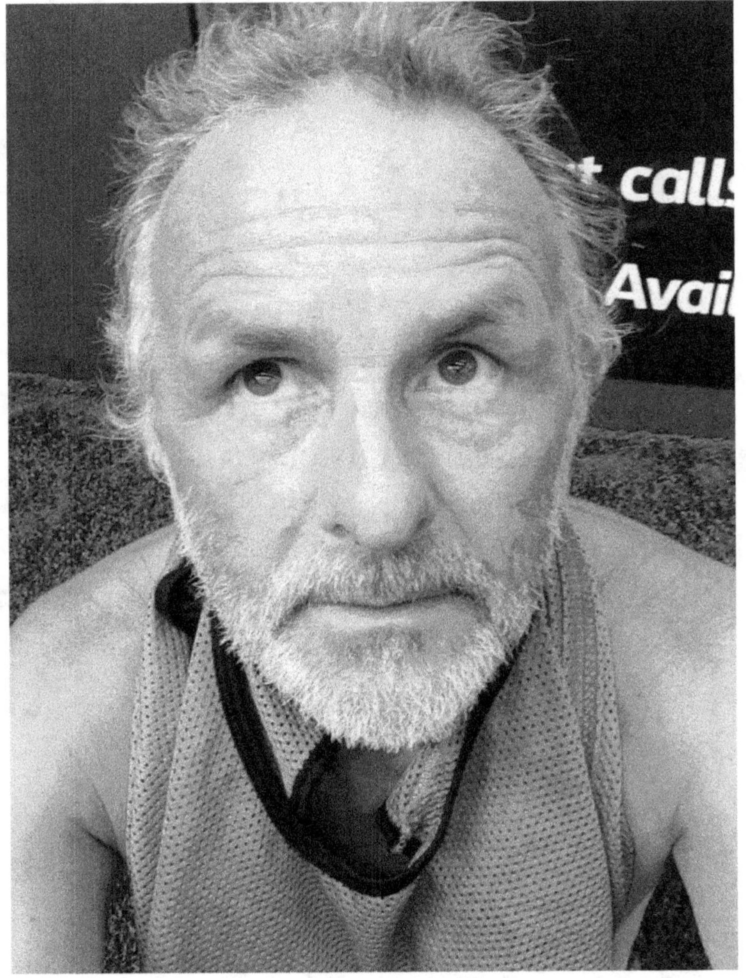

And this is me now!!!

Tatty bye, then.

ACKNOWLEDGEMENTS

In order for me to write this book I needed a lot of peoples' help. Not with the writing, setting out or putting together, but with all its contents. Without their help this book wouldn't have been possible.

On getting me here from the moment I knew what was going on, the only complaint I have is to the driver on the 38 bus.

But a very special thanks goes to this little lady, the beautiful Yvette.

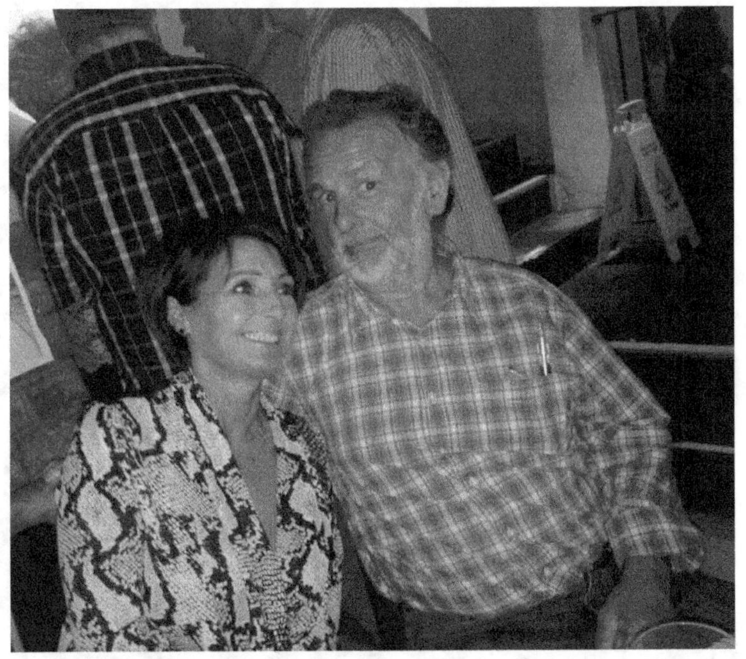

I'm punching above nothing! Shut it!

OK, so I am... And?

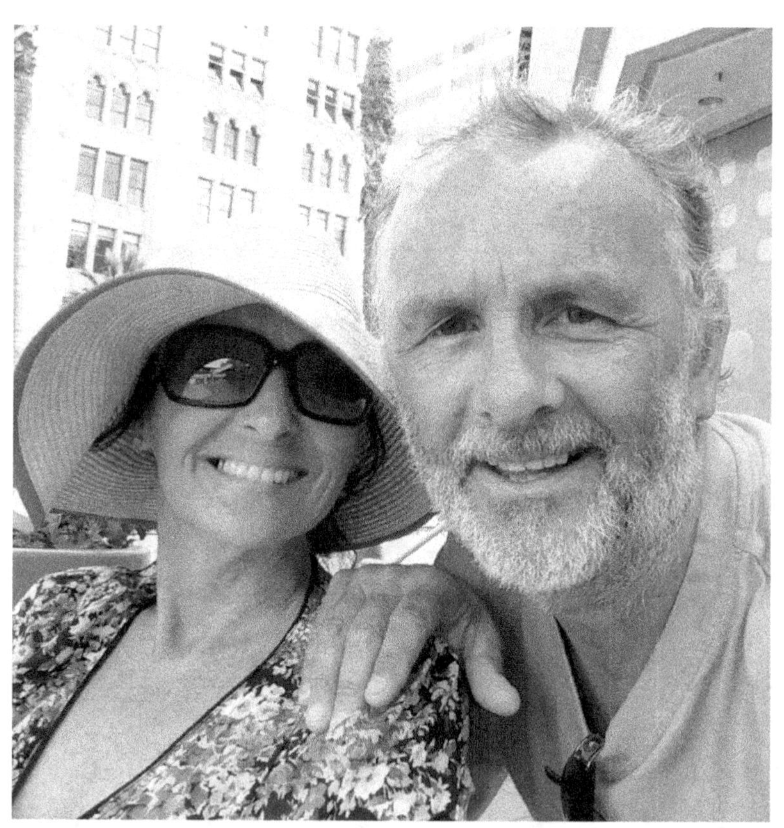

Me and Yvette.

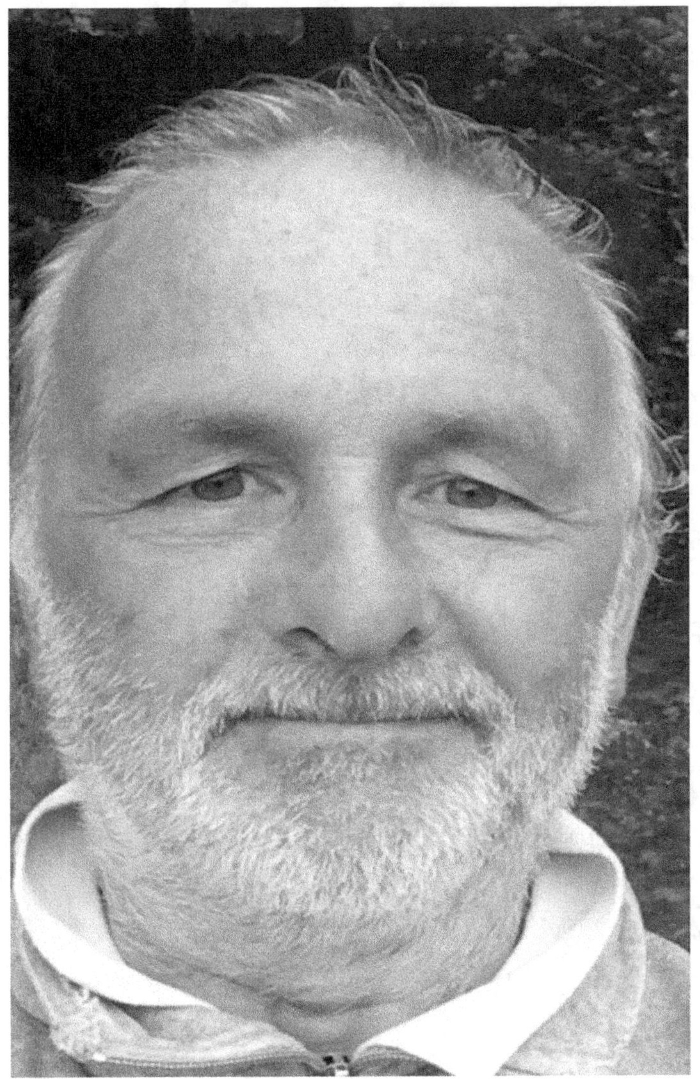

Me in 2018.

ILLUSTRATIONS AND CREDITS

All the photos used in this title were retaken by Allan Birkin for use in this book. Some of the original sources are unknown so please accept my apologies if you are not mentioned or we have used without your permission. Thank you so much.

Front cover: Shani Birkin Hodson
Back cover: The author, Shani, Ashley and Allan.

Special thanks to all who made a contribution... Muchas gracias.

Allan Birkin, the very amateur furrytographer, 2022.

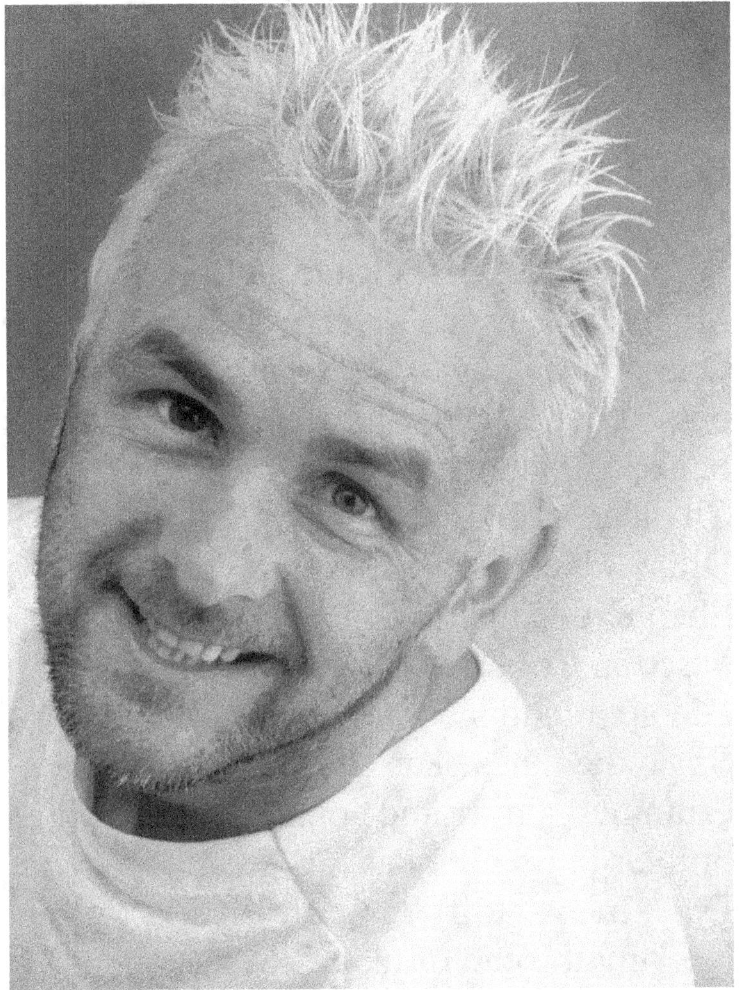

The bleached blond spikey look. Haha.

THE AUTHOR

Allan David Birkin,
Born 18th September, 1960,
Lower Broughton in Salford, UK.
Lived on Gallemore Street.
Went to Blackfriars Road Junior.
Moved to Lower Kersal.
One year of Lower Kersal Junior School,
passed the 11 Plus and went to
Salford Grammar School.
Changed to Buile Hill High School.
Did a joinery apprenticeship with
Shepperd Construction
based in Cornbrook, Manchester.
Did six months with Salford Council.
Since then, has been self-employed as a
drummer, singer and comic, as well as a
builder during the day.
Done many a different role on TV.
Nearing the end of his fifties he
is choosing to put pen to paper.
End of...

DISCLAIMER

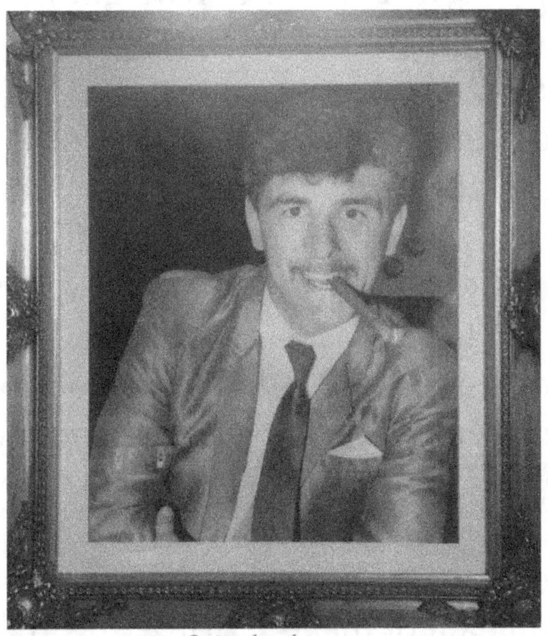

Quite the charmer.

If things are not as they seem or not as they should be then please accept my apologies. As for all my quotes and photographs, if I've used one or two that didn't belong to me, again I apologise wholeheartedly.

Love you all xxxxx

Special thanks over the years go to Arthur Waite and Jim Cartwright (photographers), Harry Barnes, Henry Harrison, Allan Guest and all the agents who put bread and butter on my dinner table, all the acts and musicians I worked with, male and female strippers I watched haha, the roadies that kept my journeys sane, the landlords, landladies and committee members that let me perform at their venues, and last (but by no means least) all family and friends xxxxx

They say you can take a horse to water but you cannot make it drink. In simple layman's terms, don't ask me to borrow one of my books so you can read it. You probably won't read it, but if you go ahead and purchase it from Amazon and it cost you dollars. you're more likely to read it. Drink up, people!

ITEMS FOR SALE

Missed the Boat
Last Day Back in the Room

Coming soon:
Why Are We Here?
The next big thing
The screenplay

Please email adb180960@hotmail.com
with any enquiries.

"A Member's Tale" is a section in The Ticker Club's quarterly magazine that features members who have gone through a heart procedure. The following was my article for the magazine. We include it unedited. Thank you.

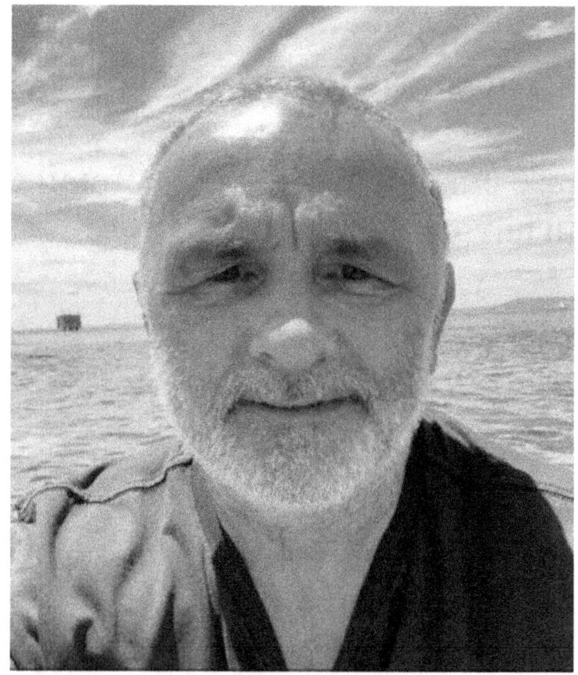

Allan again.

A MEMBER'S TALE

ALLAN BIRKIN

3 years after my story began ive just made a return visit to ward f6 on arrival i bumped into the same friendly little man still volunteering for the ticker club who was politely going about his business of re assurance offering help and advice , i was there to visit my cousin 5 years my junior almost the 8th of our family members to endure heart problems he was due to undergo a triple by pass .

I consider myself as very lucky, although i wasn't plagued with illness , at 53 years old, i got a little pre warning all wasn't right with my heart, as it turned out i had a leaky valve , and so began the process that 18 mths later led me to my 13 day stay in wythenshawe hospital i had my leaky valve replaced with a mechanical one. Although not totally full of bounce and the joys of spring i do feel blessed to still be treading these boards , i do however forget im a lot closer to 60 than the age i still think and feel i am , 21.

I became a ticker club member immediatley after i left hospital but i had made my mind up to both become a member and give a little back . My inspiration came from the very first friday afternoon meeting before my operation, where id met mike brown . He was the physiotherapist giving a talk as part of the reabilitation team , he was great , both funny and charming and the ultimate profesional , i decided in my own way i would do something that would not only give back once but have the potential and possibility to give back time and time again and better still keep on giving long after im gone . I wrote a christmas song and recorded several different versions with the help of a group of friends under the group name of "the xmas club" that will be available on line from september onwards on tune core and itunes all of the profits raised will make there way into the ticker clubs coffers . My next one is a book which will be available on amazon it's a book entitled " last day – back in the room" it tells the tale of my experience from discovering i had a leaky valve to the operating table and onwards into my future after the operation, a good insight wether music be your thing or reading please choose one or both and help me to help you to help them thank you Allan Birkin

ALSO AVAILABLE:
MISSED THE BOAT

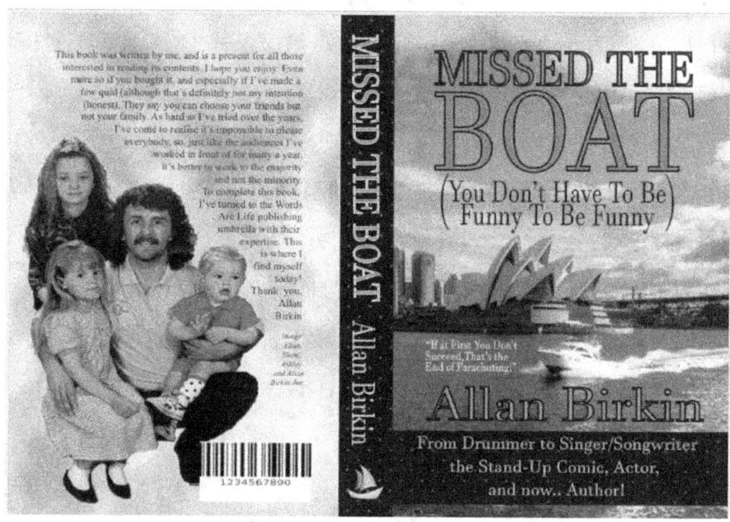

Cover of Missed the Boat.

From drummer to singer to stand-up comedian missed the boat tells the story of that marvellous journey and the realisation that if I carried on another fifty years, I still wouldn't reach the pinnacle of TV and live entertainment.

COMING SOON

Why Are We Here? The Next Big Thing

SCREENPLAY

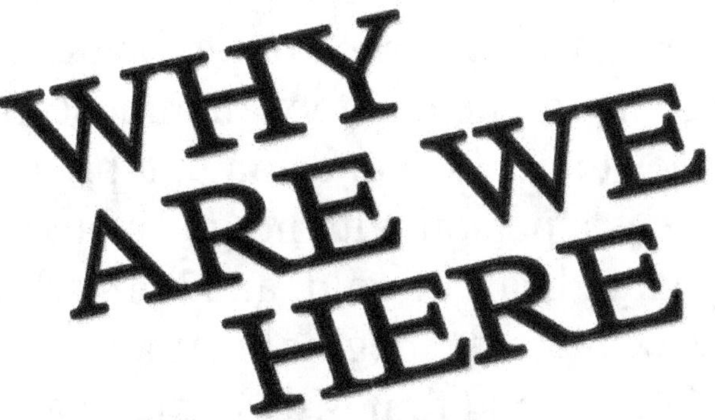

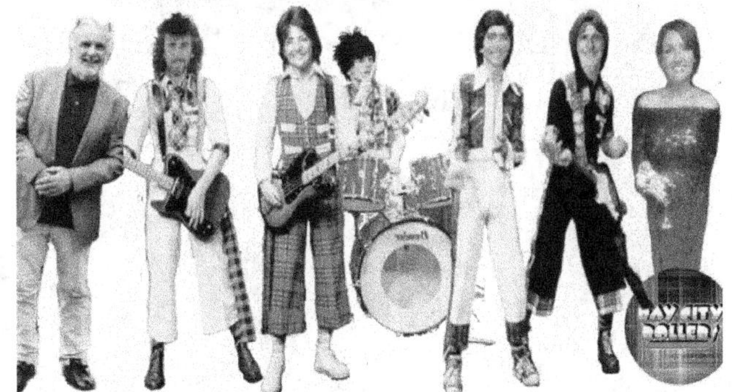

ALLAN BIRKIN 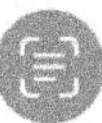

SYNOPSIS

From the moment he was born, right up to the present day, Allan's goal has been to find or invent the next big thing. As it happens, Yvette turned out to be his big thing, though he had to wait almost four decades to get his hands on that prize. Yvette is a person with no goals but a very large heart of gold, and both she and Allan witness the beginning, the duration, and (as all good things do come to an end), the decline of the biggest thing to happen in pop in the 1970s, the Scottish pop phenomenon, The Bay City Rollers.

COMMENTS

Feel free to write your own comments here and forward to adb180960@hotmail.com.

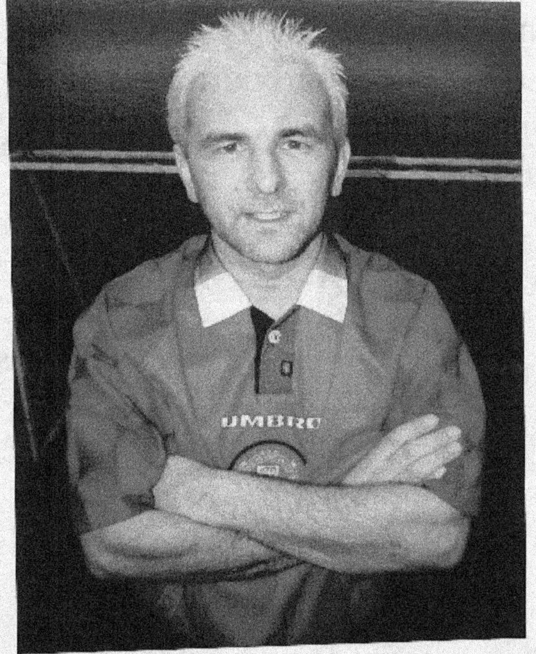

A final goodbye, and thanks for reading.

One of the good things about life is when you get something wrong, you have the opportunity to put it right. This is a blessing. In my first book, *Missed the Boat*, there were a few issues with two photographs that I spread across two pages. They didn't turn out how I wanted so here is my chance to show the photos how I wanted to show them.

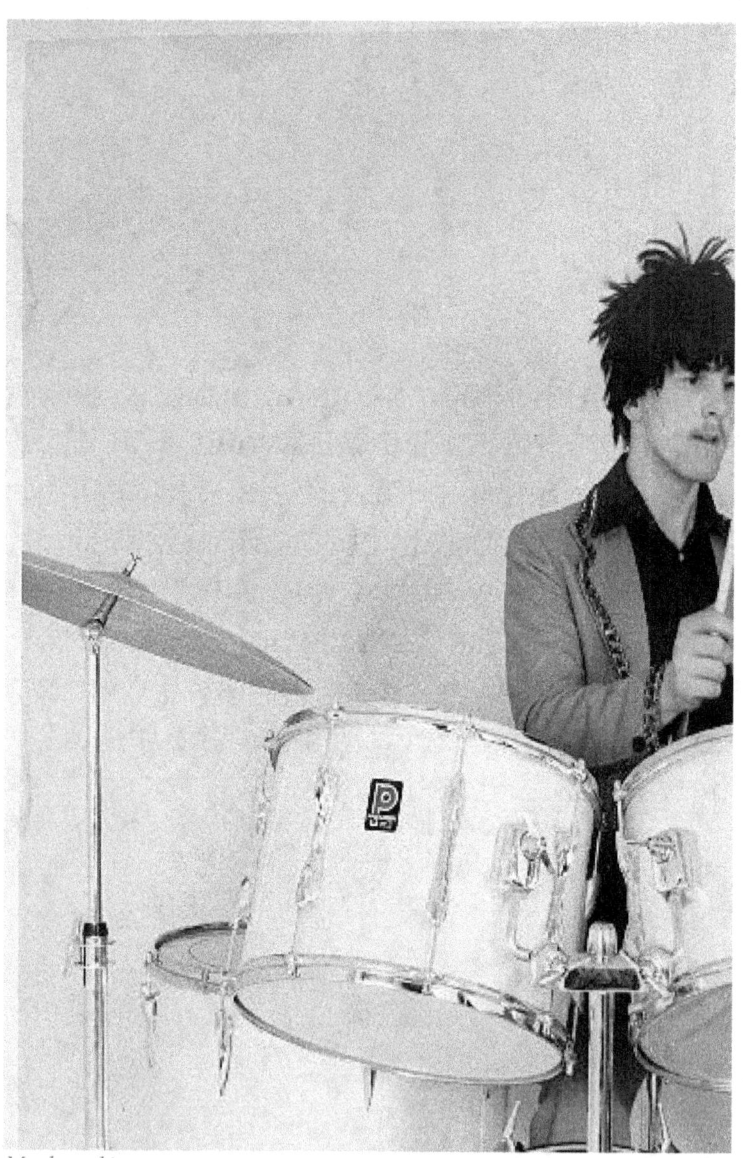

My drum kit.

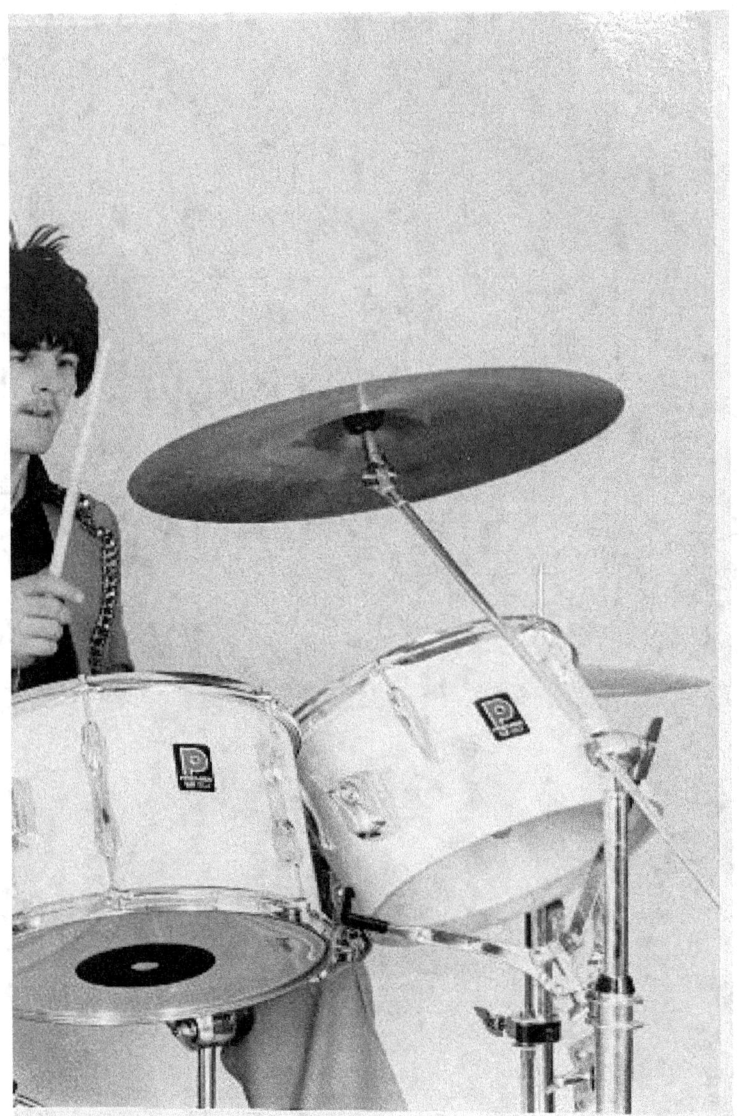

My drum kit.

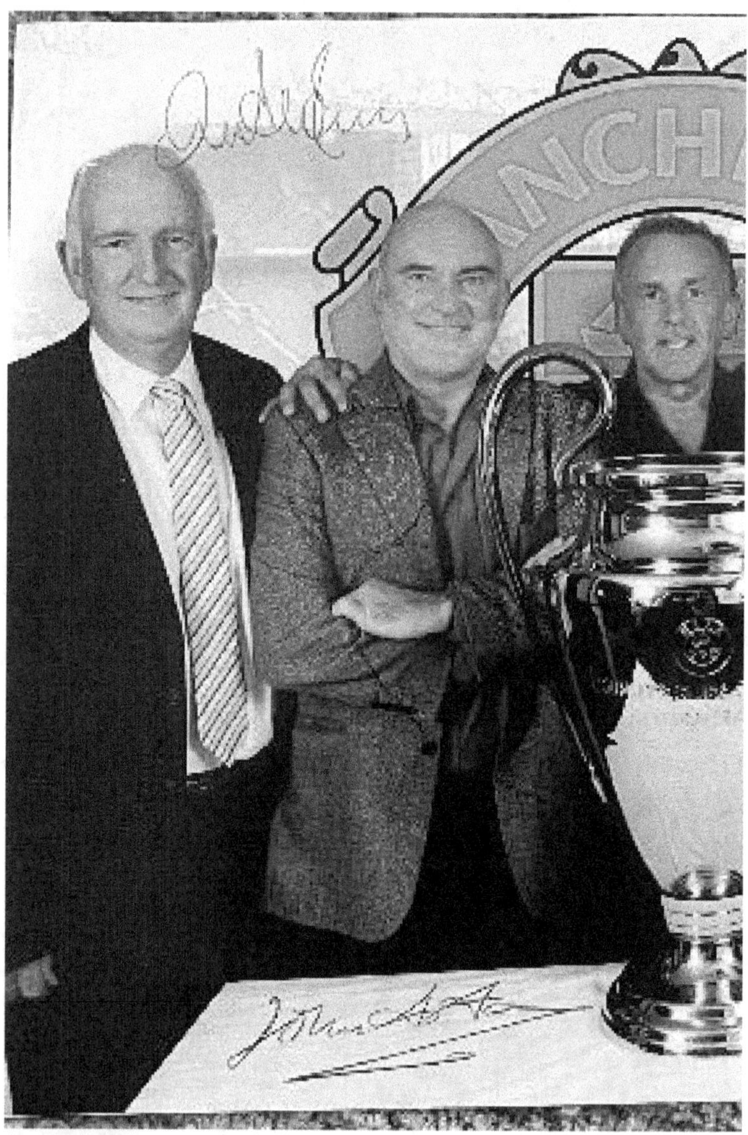

Some of my favourite footballers!

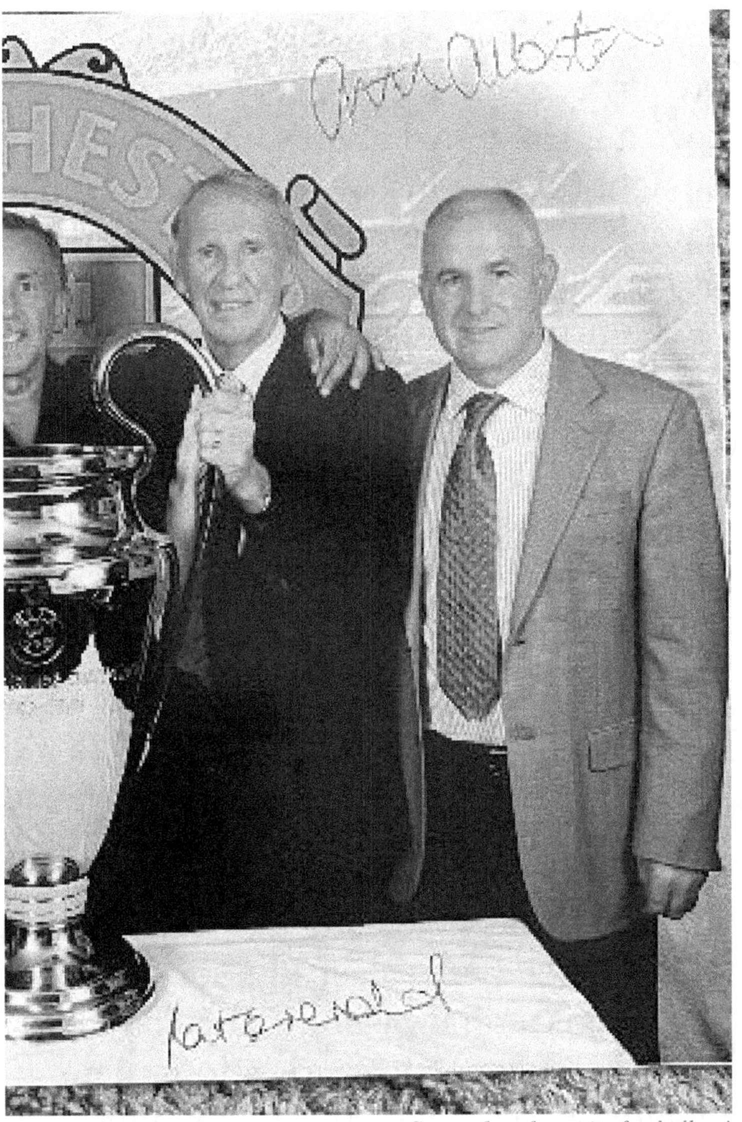

Some of my favourite footballers!

The 2nd photo is of some of my favourite ex-footballers, so, because I have a great vested interest in football, I thought I'd mention two rules I came up with. I'm still attempting to get the FA to listen to them!

The first rule – when a team scores a goal, in their rush to get the ball back to the centre spot, the team members of the team that's just conceded withhold the ball in a delaying tactic, resulting in a bit of argy bargy that very often gets out of hand.

A simple remedy to eliminate this type of action would be to make it a yellow card offence for any member of the conceding team to touch the ball – unless the scoring team walk away with no desire to collect the ball.

The second rule is substitutions. Subbing is a timewasting tactic that infuriates a losing team. Sergio Agüero would run his socks off for 85 minutes then when he was substituted would all of a sudden discover there was broken glass in his boots. He would walk off accordingly. My answer was that, when they make a substitution, the game should carry on. The substitute cannot enter the field of play until the substituted player has left the pitch, and, if he touches the ball before leaving the pitch it is a red card offence. This means that not only does the substitute not come on but the substituted player will exit that pitch at an astronomical speed.

www.ingramcontent.com/pod-product-compliance
Lightning Source LLC
Chambersburg PA
CBHW061600250726
48657CB00020B/65